THE 14-DAY ELIMINATION DIET PLAN

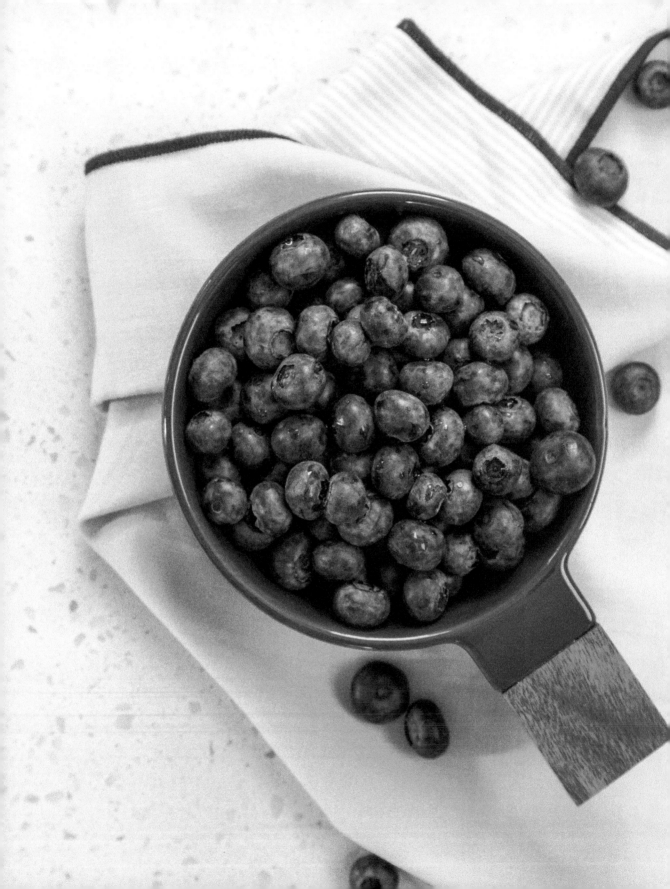

THE 14-DAY
Elimination
Diet Plan

Identify Food Allergies and Sensitivities the No-Stress Way

Tara Rochford, RDN

ROCKRIDGE
PRESS

For general information on our other products and services or to obtain technical support, please contact our Customer Care Department within the U.S. at (866) 744-2665, or outside the U.S. at (510) 253-0500.

Rockridge Press publishes its books in a variety of electronic and print formats. Some content that appears in print may not be available in electronic books, and vice versa.

Interior and Cover Designer: Lisa Forde
Art Producer: Michael Hardgrove
Editor: Pam Kingsley
Production Editor: Andrew Yackira and Claire Yee

Photography © 2019 Amy Johnson, Food styling by Rachel Grunig, cover, and pp. ii, vi, x, 24, 26, 56, 58, 66, 94, 106, 130, 150, 164. Photography © Marija Vidal, pp. ix, 12; Shannon Douglas, p. 2; Nadine Greeff, p. 20; Shannon Douglas, p. 46; Author photo courtesy of © Kelley Jordan Schuyler.

ISBN: Print 978-1-64152-686-9 |
        eBook 978-1-64152-687-6

To Brian, my wonderful husband,
biggest fan, and best friend.

To my mom, who knows me better than I know
myself and always has the right thing to say.

To my favorite pups, Bernie and Rooney, who sat on
my lap and licked every crumb as I wrote this book.

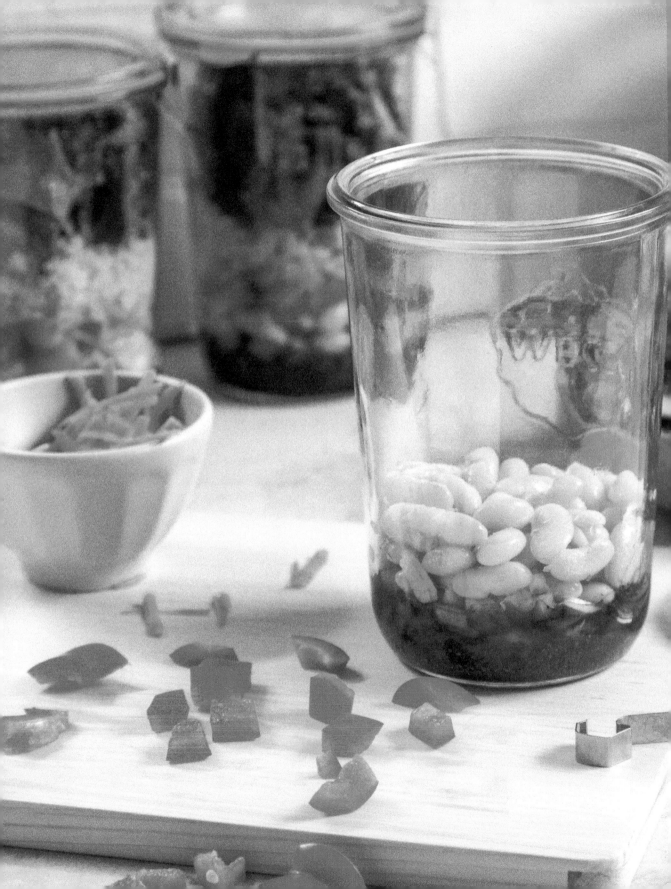

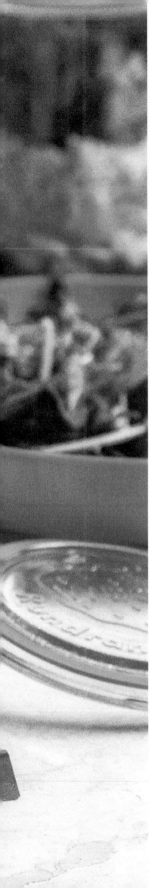

Contents

Introduction

It is my mission to share with the world that nourishing foods are delicious and comforting for the soul and should never be tasteless or bland. Part of accomplishing that mission is helping people—helping you—find the foods that allow you to be your best version of you.

As an individual diagnosed with irritable bowel syndrome (IBS) a few years ago, I understand how it feels to not know what is causing your symptoms. It can be frustrating, scary, defeating, and lonely, but know that I am here for you. While it takes work to find all the pieces of the puzzle, this book can be a tool to help you learn what foods allow you to thrive and which need to be eliminated to ensure your good health.

What Is the Elimination Diet?

Food allergies and intolerances, while different, both appear to be increasing in incidence. Food allergies affect over 30 million people in the United States and nearly 250 million people worldwide. It's unclear if the numbers are truly increasing or if there is simply more awareness of food allergies and intolerances. Either way, many people are affected by these conditions.

According to the Academy of Nutrition and Dietetics, the oral food challenge is the gold standard for diagnosing a true food allergy. In other words, the only way to know if you have an allergy to or intolerance of a food is to eat it. Through personal experience and working with clients in a one-on-one setting, I understand that eliminating foods, pinpointing trigger foods, and reintroducing foods can be extremely confusing and time-consuming.

I've developed the Elimination Diet based on the eight major allergens, plus other potentially allergenic foods and foods that may cause intolerance. This diet first removes all foods that might cause issues, then strategically reintroduces foods from each category so you can monitor your symptoms.

Many common, nutritious ingredients are eliminated temporarily during this time, but the recipes I've created are flavorful enough to share with friends and family who don't suffer from food allergies or intolerances.

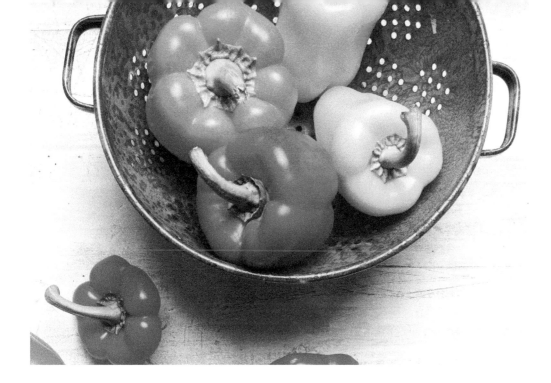

How to Use This Book

This book is yours to use. I want you to view it as a workbook. Highlight symptoms, flag pages, share recipes, and write in the journal. Doing this will help you figure out what foods are going to make you feel healthy.

The book begins by explaining what a food allergy is and describing each potential allergen as well as its symptoms, the age group most commonly affected by it, and if it will ever go away. I then discuss food intolerances and explain the details there, too. Part 1 examines the symptoms I've listed and notes where they line up with the symptoms you have been experiencing. Many food allergies produce similar symptoms, and the severity varies depending on the individual, but this is a great starting point.

After understanding what may be causing your symptoms and what other symptoms to watch for, I explain the details of the Elimination Diet, which consists of the elimination phase and the reintroduction phase. Each recipe created in this book calls for foods that should not cause a reaction (see pages 28–31). If you are taking medications, please consult your doctor about any associated dietary restrictions before beginning the Elimination Diet Plan. I want you to figure out what is causing your symptoms while enjoying delicious and satisfying food, but keep in mind that this way of eating is not forever. The goal is to help you eat and enjoy as many foods as possible.

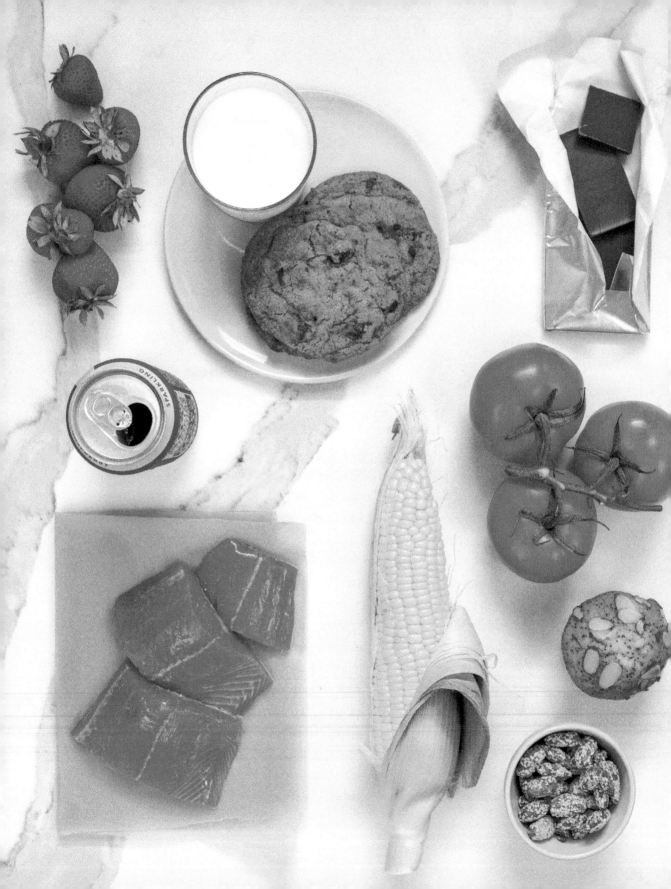

PART 1

Food Allergies and Sensitivities

FOOD ALLERGIES ARE potentially life-threatening, and food sensitivities and intolerances can be extremely uncomfortable. They can also be some of the most confusing and misunderstood conditions. While the foods listed in part 1 may be causing you distress, it's important to recognize that many of the foods causing allergies and intolerances are nutritious and healthy for people who don't react to them. This is why it's important to determine what foods you react to, and then work with a medical professional to come up with an accurate diagnosis.

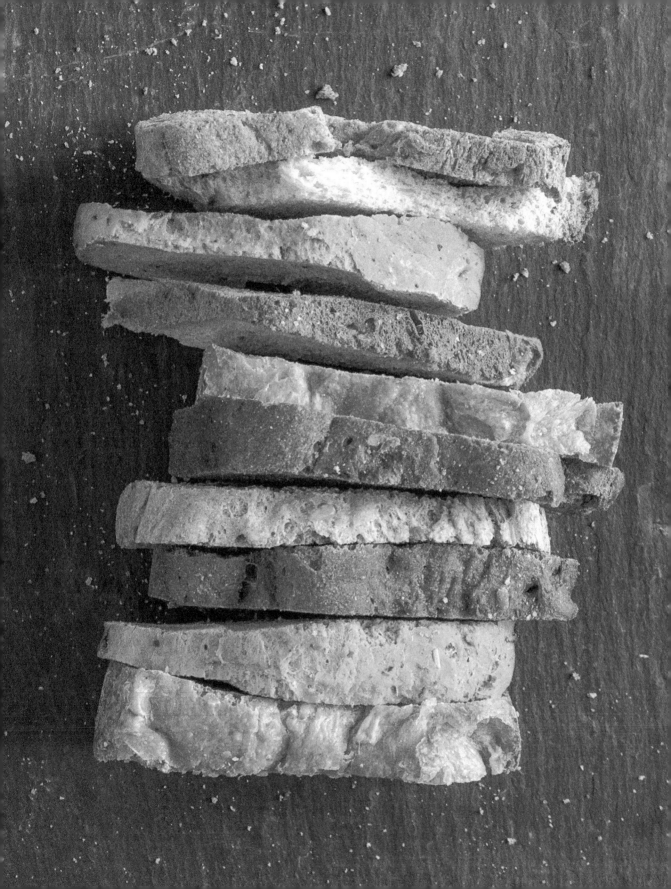

CHAPTER 1

Food Allergies

This chapter explains exactly what a food allergy is and which foods may trigger it. We'll also explore who is most susceptible to food allergies, whether people can grow out of them, and what the various symptoms might be. This will be a great place to reference as you pay attention to the symptoms you are experiencing.

What Is a Food Allergy?

A food allergy is a negative health effect caused by a specific response of the immune system that is reproducible with exposure to a given food. A reaction that occurs only sometimes when a food is eaten, or a reaction that does not include the immune system, is not a true food allergy. In this book, I mention the term *sensitization* a few times, which is the process by which the body produces a defensive protein or antibody so that future exposures to a food or allergen will produce an allergic reaction. Symptoms from a food allergy may be simply uncomfortable, or they may be life-threatening. Symptoms usually develop within a few minutes of consuming the food or up to two hours afterward. The most common food allergy symptoms are an itchy or tingling mouth; hives, itching, or eczema; swelling of the face, lips, tongue, or other body parts; wheezing; trouble breathing; stuffy nose; stomach pain; diarrhea; nausea; vomiting; dizziness; lightheadedness; fainting; and/or anaphylaxis. It is important to note that anaphylaxis is a life-threatening condition, and if you or someone you are with experiences this, you should immediately use an epinephrine shot

(EpiPen) and seek medical attention. Anaphylaxis can occur with exposure to something you are allergic to, such as peanuts, a bee sting, venom, or medication. Signs and symptoms of anaphylaxis include rapid and weak pulse, low blood pressure, skin rash, nausea, vomiting, dizziness, fainting, and constriction of your airway. You may experience one or more of these symptoms.

When you have a food allergy, your body is mistaking the food you are eating for something harmful. Your body responds in an attempt to protect you by releasing an antibody called immunoglobulin E (IgE) to help fight the allergen. The next time you eat that same food, even a very small amount, IgE antibodies sense that food and remember it as being harmful, and they fight to protect you by releasing chemicals into your body. These chemicals cause the allergic reaction.

Dairy/Cow's Milk

A dairy or cow's milk allergy is a negative immune-system response to the protein in milk or other dairy products. Consuming cow's milk is the usual cause of the reaction, but sometimes milk from other mammals (sheep, goat, buffalo) can also provoke it. These allergies are most common in early childhood, and many children will outgrow them.

Symptoms of a milk allergy occur within a few minutes to a few hours after consuming the milk or food containing milk. Symptoms that may show up right away include hives; wheezing; itching or tingling in the mouth, lips, or throat; swelling of the mouth, lips, tongue, or throat; coughing; and/or vomiting. Symptoms that may take a few hours to develop are diarrhea that may contain blood, stomach cramping or pain, runny nose, watery eyes, and colic in babies. Milk allergy can also cause life-threatening anaphylaxis.

If you or your child experience an allergic reaction or any of these symptoms after consuming milk or milk products, it is important to talk to your doctor or an allergist to create an accurate diagnosis.

A dairy or cow's milk allergy is different from lactose intolerance, which does not involve the immune system. You can read more about lactose intolerance on page 15.

Wheat

Wheat allergy is one of the most common allergies in Western countries and is most typically seen in children, though most will outgrow the condition over time. Adults can also be diagnosed with wheat allergies, though this is less common.

The protein in wheat causes the immune system response and food allergy. Wheat proteins include four classes: gliadins, glutenins, albumins, and globulins. No single protein or class of protein appears to be responsible for a wheat allergy.

Symptoms of a wheat allergy vary with the individual. Some people develop symptoms only if they exercise within a few hours of eating wheat. This is called food-dependent exercise-induced anaphylaxis (FDEIA); see page 10. Other symptoms will develop within minutes or a few hours of consumption and include swelling, itching, or irritation of the throat or mouth, hives, itchy rash, skin swelling, stuffy nose, headache, difficulty breathing, cramps, nausea, vomiting, diarrhea, and/or life-threatening anaphylaxis.

Celiac disease and wheat allergies are different conditions. The gluten in wheat, rye, and barley causes celiac disease. The type of antibody involved in celiac disease is immunoglobulin A (IgA) rather than IgE, which is what is involved in a wheat allergy. You can read more about celiac disease on page 15.

Eggs

Egg allergy is one of the most common food allergies in children, but most children outgrow it. Symptoms of an egg allergy typically happen within a few minutes to a few hours after something containing egg has been eaten and can include skin rashes or hives; stuffy or runny nose and sneezing; digestive issues like cramps, nausea, or vomiting; symptoms similar to asthma, like wheezing and difficulty breathing; and/or life-threatening anaphylaxis. Proteins in egg yolks and whites can cause an allergic reaction, so susceptible individuals are advised to avoid egg in any form.

Many food labels state "may contain egg" or "manufactured in a facility that also processes egg," but it is still extremely important to be aware of foods that may contain egg but are not labeled.

Fish

Finned fish allergy is most common among adults and is usually lifelong. If you have an allergy to finned fish (salmon, tuna, cod, etc.), it does not necessarily mean you have an allergy to shellfish (muscles, shrimp, crab, etc.). Some individuals may have a reaction to only one kind of finned fish. More research is needed in this area, so it is very important to work with your physician or allergist to come up with a plan that addresses your specific allergy.

Allergic reactions from fish are usually caused by the muscle (flesh) and collagen, which is contained in the skin and bones. Fish protein may be found in wine or beer due to the use of isinglass, a type of gelatin that comes from the air bladders of certain fish and is used to clarify wine or beer. If you think you may have a fish allergy, it is important to avoid beer and wine that undergo this filtering method. African, Indonesian, Chinese, Thai, and Vietnamese cuisines all have a high risk of finned fish presence because of their use of ingredients like fish sauce. Before consuming these cuisines, be sure to inquire about their contents.

Fish allergies can cause a life-threatening anaphylactic response in addition to other symptoms such as hives, skin rash, nausea, stomach cramps, diarrhea, vomiting, stuffy or runny nose, sneezing, headaches, and/or asthma.

Shellfish

Shellfish allergy is caused by the body's immune system responding to proteins in crustaceans (crab, lobster, crawfish, shrimp/prawns), mollusks (oysters, mussels, clams), and cephalopods (squid and octopus). Some people react to all shellfish, and some people react to only certain kinds. If you experience symptoms when eating shellfish, talk with your doctor or allergist so you can get an accurate diagnosis. African, Indonesian, Chinese, Thai, and Vietnamese cuisines all have a high risk of shellfish presence because of their use of ingredients like shrimp paste. Before consuming these cuisines, be sure to inquire about their contents.

Anyone at any age can develop a shellfish allergy, but it is more common in adults. Symptoms of a shellfish allergy may develop in as little as a few minutes or up to an hour after a food is eaten. Symptoms include hives, itchy skin, or eczema; swelling of the lips, face, tongue, throat, or other parts of the body; wheezing or difficulty breathing; stuffy nose; stomach pain, nausea, vomiting, or diarrhea; dizziness; fainting; and life-threatening anaphylaxis.

Soybeans and Soy Products

Soy allergy commonly develops in infancy and can often be discovered through a reaction to soy-based formula. Most children outgrow soy allergies, but some maintain them throughout adulthood.

Symptoms include hives; itching or tingling around the mouth; eczema; swelling of the lips, face, tongue, or other body parts; wheezing; runny nose; difficulty breathing; stomach pain; diarrhea; vomiting; skin redness; and/or life-threatening anaphylaxis.

Soy allergy may also cause a delayed allergic response called food protein–induced enterocolitis syndrome (FPIES). In this case, vomiting and nausea occur hours after eating the soy product.

Peanuts

Peanut allergy is one of the most common causes of life-threatening allergy attacks. If anaphylaxis occurs, it is a medical emergency. For some people with a peanut allergy, even a very small amount can cause a dangerous reaction.

Peanuts contain many different proteins, and several of these can trigger IgE antibodies to cause an allergic reaction. As with other allergies, symptoms vary between individuals. Commonly seen symptoms are hives, red skin, swelling around the lips and face, wheezing, noisy breathing, coughing, throat tightening, stuffy nose, asthma, vomiting, diarrhea, stomach pain, low blood pressure, irregular heartbeat, and/or life-threatening anaphylaxis.

If you or your child experiences any kind of reaction to peanuts, it is important to talk with your doctor or allergist. Allergic reactions can be unpredictable—while an individual might experience only mild symptoms at first, they may still be at risk for far more serious reactions in the future.

Most peanut allergies appear to last a lifetime, but some children can outgrow them. When this happens, individuals are encouraged to consume peanuts regularly as part of a nutritious diet.

Be aware that African, Chinese, Indonesian, Mexican, Thai, and Vietnamese cuisines all have a high risk for cross-contamination even if you order a peanut-free dish.

Tree Nuts

Tree nut allergies can occur in children and adults and often last a lifetime. Peanuts are legumes and are botanically unrelated to tree nuts such as walnuts, pecans, Brazil nuts, almonds, cashews, hazelnuts, macadamia nuts, pine nuts, chestnuts, and so on. While some people have allergic reactions to coconut, it is not a botanical nut, so having a tree nut allergy does not automatically mean you have a coconut allergy. Many people who are allergic to tree nuts can still eat peanuts and coconut, so in order to enjoy as many foods as possible, it is important to manage your allergies with a medical professional.

This allergy may lead to an anaphylactic response, so it is very important that individuals who are allergic to tree nuts be aware of the ingredients they are consuming as well as of potential cross-contamination.

Other possible symptoms include stomach pain, cramps, nausea, vomiting, or diarrhea; difficulty swallowing; itchy mouth, throat, eyes, or skin; stuffy or runny nose; and/or shortness of breath.

Sesame

Sesame (also known as benne) is a flowering plant producing edible seeds that are used in many dishes from bagel toppings to sushi. Current US guidelines do not require the use of sesame to be labeled by food manufacturers, as it is not one of the top eight food allergens, but research shows that an increasing number of individuals have sesame allergies.

This allergy can develop at any age. When looking at the structure of most plants, the most highly allergenic molecules are associated with storage proteins (also known as albumins) in the seed. This part of the plant may have defense mechanisms to protect the plant and help with reproduction. Even though the protein is what typically causes the allergic response, individuals should also avoid use of sesame oil. Most people with a sesame allergy do not have other seed allergies.

Symptoms may include headache, hives, swelling, difficulty breathing, diarrhea, nausea, vomiting, loss of consciousness, anxiety, and/or life-threatening anaphylaxis.

Corn

Allergic reactions to corn can be caused by an individual being sensitized to corn, corn protein, or corn pollen. This may be challenging to navigate because corn and corn products are used in the process of creating many foods and products.

As ingredients such as high-fructose corn syrup do not contain corn protein, they may not be allergenic to individuals with a corn allergy, though it is best to discuss this detail with your doctor or allergist to avoid having a dangerous reaction.

Symptoms of a corn allergy may show up a few minutes or a few hours after consumption and can include vomiting, stomach cramps, or diarrhea; wheezing or difficulty breathing; coughing or throat tightening; weak pulse; pale or blue skin; hives; swelling of the lips, face, tongue, or other body parts; dizziness; confusion; and/or life-threatening anaphylaxis.

Pollen-Food Allergy Syndrome

Pollen-food allergy syndrome, also known as oral allergy syndrome (OAS), is caused by reactions from allergens found in pollen, raw fruits, some vegetables, and some tree nuts. This occurs because the protein in some fruit, vegetables, and tree nuts is very similar to the protein in pollen. When the allergenic food is eaten, the body recognizes the pollen or similar protein in the food and signals the body to have an allergic response. Because cooking denatures proteins (meaning it disrupts or even destroys their structure), many people with OAS can consume cooked versions of the fruits they are allergic to.

This allergy typically does not appear in young children. It is usually seen in teens, young adults, and older adults who have consumed the allergenic food previously many times without any reaction. Individuals with OAS typically have allergies to birch, ragweed, or grass pollens.

Symptoms of OAS usually appear immediately after consuming the allergenic food but can sometimes take up to an hour to appear. They include a scratchy mouth or throat, swollen lips or areas around the mouth, itchy ears, and/or hives. Anaphylaxis is a rare reaction.

Latex-Fruit Allergy

Natural rubber latex is made of proteins that may cause an allergic reaction in certain individuals. Some foods that are completely unrelated to latex-producing trees contain proteins that have almost the same structure as the proteins found in latex. When people who are allergic to latex come into contact with or eat these foods, an allergic reaction occurs. This condition is called latex-fruit allergy, but other foods besides fruit may cause a reaction.

An estimated 50 to 70 percent of people with latex allergies have IgE antibodies that may cross-react with proteins in certain plant foods, but it's important to remember that all individuals with latex allergies react differently to foods with cross-reacting proteins. Not everyone with a latex allergy has allergic reactions to fruits, and those who do may not react to the same fruits. Symptoms may range from a mild allergic reaction to life-threatening anaphylaxis.

Food-Dependent Exercise-Induced Anaphylaxis

Exercise-induced allergies are most commonly seen in adults. Individuals with FDEIA experience symptoms such as lightheadedness, itchiness, or life-threatening anaphylaxis shortly after they start exercising. Different foods cause this reaction in different people, so it is hard to list which foods to avoid. If you experience these symptoms, avoid consuming food at least two hours prior to physical activity, avoid consuming foods that can cause this reaction, and see your doctor or allergist to come up with a diagnosis management plan that works for you.

Meat Allergy

The meat from any mammal, such as beef, lamb, pork, goat, whale, and seal, has the potential to cause an allergic reaction. This is an uncommon condition, but if you experience a stuffy nose, develop a rash, or feel nauseated after consuming meat, you may have a meat allergy.

This allergy can develop at any stage of life, and if you are allergic to one kind of meat, it is likely you are allergic to other kinds of meat.

Symptoms include hives, skin rash, nausea, stomach pain or cramps, diarrhea, vomiting, stuffy or runny nose, sneezing, headaches, asthma, or life-threatening anaphylaxis. It is important to note that while an anaphylactic reaction to most allergenic foods is immediate, in the case of a meat allergy, this reaction may be delayed for several hours after meat consumption. Many times, the development of a meat allergy can be traced back to getting bitten by a Lone Star tick.

If you suspect that you may be suffering from a meat allergy, it is important to avoid the food(s) you are reacting to and consult with an allergist.

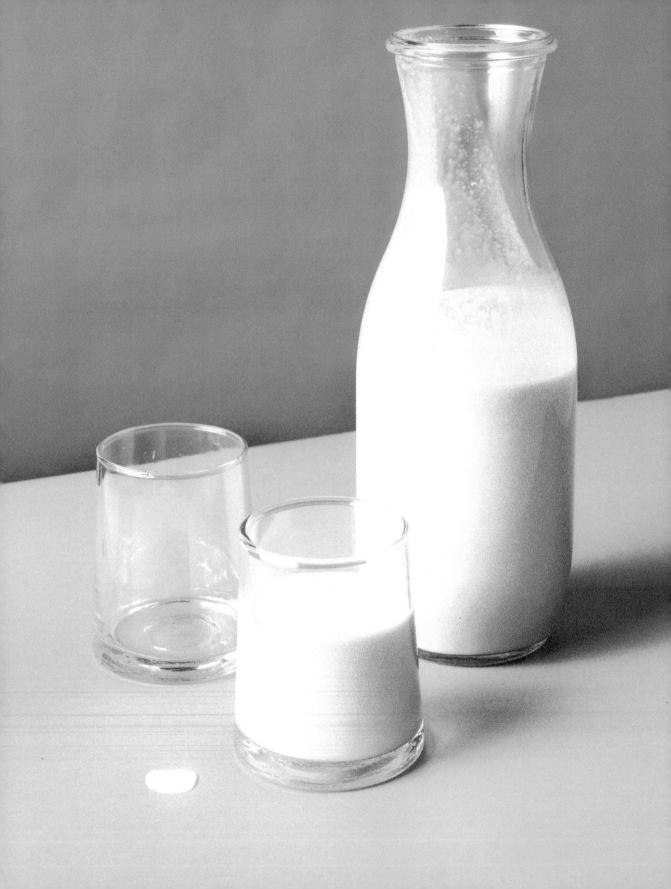

CHAPTER 2

Food Intolerances and Sensitivities

In this chapter, we'll dig into food intolerances and sensitivities and explain the difference in how the body reacts to a food intolerance versus a food allergy. Then we'll take a look at many common food intolerances and the foods that may be causing your symptoms.

What Is a Food Sensitivity/Intolerance?

A food sensitivity or intolerance is an adverse reaction to food that results from the way the body digests the food. Symptoms of a food intolerance may resemble those of a food allergy and may include bloating, gas, diarrhea, stomach pain, constipation, nausea, low energy, migraines, hives, rash, and/or eczema.

There are several potential causes of food intolerances, including enzyme deficiencies, gastrointestinal diseases, sensitivity to food additives, reactions to naturally occurring chemicals in food, neurological issues, or metabolic conditions individuals are born with.

As we saw in chapter 1, immunoglobulin E (IgE) responses, such as hives or anaphylactic reactions, are immediate, may be life-threatening, and are true food allergies. The immune reaction found in food intolerances, by contrast, is mediated by immunoglobulin A (IgA), which is an antibody found in our mucous membranes that helps us fight bacteria, viruses, and other environmental toxins. Sometimes, however, IgA reactions occur when we consume certain foods. IgA reactions have a delayed response, and when we are sensitive to a certain food, it may take hours or days for us to feel the effects.

Gluten

Gluten is a general name for a certain protein found in wheat, barley, rye, and triticale (a cross between wheat and rye). Gluten acts as a glue in these foods to help maintain their shape; it can also be found in many foods as a food additive. Oats are naturally gluten-free and can provide variety and nutrition benefits to those following a gluten-free diet, but cross-contamination may occur in many processing facilities. Because of this, if you have celiac disease, non-celiac gluten sensitivity, or another condition that limits your ability to tolerate gluten, it is important to purchase oats that are labeled "certified gluten-free."

CELIAC DISEASE

Celiac disease is a serious autoimmune condition caused by an adverse reaction to certain foods and is mediated by the immune system, but it is not an IgE-mediated reaction.

When someone with celiac disease eats gluten, their body responds by attacking parts of the small intestine. Under a microscope, the villi of the small intestine appear flattened and distorted, which is an important part of diagnosing someone with celiac disease.

People at any age can be diagnosed with celiac disease, and it is important for long-term health to receive a diagnosis as soon as possible. Symptoms include bloating, brain fog, stomach pain, diarrhea, stool containing fat (it floats in the water), weight loss, fatigue, anemia, vomiting, and/or poor appetite.

GLUTEN INTOLERANCE

People with non-celiac gluten sensitivity (NCGS) experience similar symptoms to people with celiac disease, but they do not test positive for celiac disease. These symptoms improve when gluten is removed from their diet.

A recent study compared healthy individuals with people who have celiac disease and NCGS and found that the individuals with NCGS experience a body-wide inflammatory immune response possibly due to a weakened intestinal barrier. While more research is needed in this area, this study shows that the symptoms people with NCGS experience are not imagined, as many once thought.

Lactose

Lactose is the major sugar in the milk of all mammals. Lactose intolerance is caused by a lack of the digestive enzyme lactase, which breaks apart lactose into glucose and galactose. Symptoms are caused by undigested lactose in the large intestine. Many adults have a degree of lactase deficiency due to a natural decrease in the production of the enzyme.

Sometimes, it can be hard to tell the difference between milk allergies (see page 4) and lactose intolerance, because some of the symptoms are very similar. However, milk allergies often cause symptoms in areas of the body other than the digestive system, such as a runny or stuffy nose and skin reactions. It is important to determine the true cause of your symptoms by working with a doctor or allergist, because if you are reacting to lactose intolerance rather than a milk allergy, there are many dairy products that contain minimal or no lactose that you should still be able to consume.

Nitrates/Nitrites

Nitrates and nitrites are food additives used as preservatives to protect against botulism as well as to give flavor and color to manufactured foods. Nitrates are naturally occurring in many vegetables and fruits, but the level varies depending on the conditions of the soil the plants are grown in, the time of year, and the location.

Individuals' tolerance to nitrates and nitrites varies, which makes it hard to give recommendations for serving sizes and daily limits. If you think you may be sensitive to nitrates or nitrites, completing the Elimination Diet with the challenge phase outlined on page 52 will help you identify foods you are most sensitive to. Symptoms for nitrate and nitrite intolerance include anemia, difficulty breathing, pale skin, dizziness, and/or headaches.

Histamines

Histamine is a chemical released by cells in the immune system to fight foreign invaders when allergens, bacteria, illnesses, or viruses enter the body. Histamines can cause watery eyes, swelling, itching, and sneezing. If you experience seasonal allergies with these symptoms, you have firsthand experience with histamine doing its job.

Many foods and drinks contain histamine or cause the body to produce histamine. When the body is unable to break down histamine quickly enough, it ends up with more than it needs. This can result in an intolerance or sensitivity to histamine in some people. Symptoms are unpleasant and may resemble an allergic reaction.

MSG

Monosodium glutamate (MSG) is a traditional flavor enhancer in Asian cooking that is also increasingly used in Western foods. It is commonly listed as the cause of symptoms such as headache, muscle pain, backache, neck pain, nausea, unusual sweating, tingling, red face, and chest heaviness. Despite many anecdotal links between these symptoms and MSG consumption, studies conflict with regard to whether there is a scientific correlation. As a result, the reason MSG may cause symptoms in some individuals remains unknown. There are several proposed theories, but in this case, it is best to pay attention to foods that cause you to have symptoms. If you find that foods containing added MSG and natural glutamate are causing discomfort, work with your physician to come up with a tolerance threshold that works for you.

Sulfites

Sulfites are used as preservatives in packaged snack foods, prepared and presliced foods, drinks, fruits, and vegetables. They have been used for centuries and are currently the most versatile food additive in the food manufacturing industry.

Sulfite sensitivity is most common in people with asthma, and asthmatic individuals who are dependent on steroids are at the highest risk for sulfite sensitivity. Consuming sulfites may cause difficulty breathing, digestive issues, skin reactions, feeling of temperature change, swallowing difficulty, and/or symptoms in the mucous membranes. People with asthma may experience an anaphylactic reaction, but this is very rare. People with kidney or liver damage are advised to avoid consuming sulfites because there are not enough enzymes in their kidneys and liver to break down the sulfites. These people will experience symptoms of sulfite sensitivity. Sulfates do not produce the same symptoms as sulfites and don't need to be avoided.

Benzoates

Benzoates are chemicals used in a variety of manufactured food products to keep food free from contaminating microorganisms, maintain food color, and prevent water and oil from separating. Benzoates also occur naturally in some foods such as prunes, tea, cinnamon, and certain kinds of berries. While benzoates are safe for most people to consume, a small number of people have negative reactions, resulting in a range of symptoms that look similar to an allergy, including asthma, hives, swelling of the skin, stuffy nose, eczema, contact dermatitis, cutaneous vasculitis, and/or headaches. While benzoate sensitivity is not an allergy, it may make an existing allergy worse.

Artificial Colors

You may have heard the saying, "We eat with our eyes." This is why the color of food is so important in the food production industry. To obtain the most appealing color, various manufactured colors are added to common foods we eat.

Most colors used in foods are listed on the FDA's Generally Recognized as Safe (GRAS) list and have not had negative reactions associated with them. Some colors have been linked with symptoms such as hives, asthma, aspirin intolerance, itching, stuffy and runny nose, blurry vision, purple skin patches, and/or migraines. Several food dyes with the preservative benzoate have also been linked to hyperactivity in children, though more evidence is needed in this area. Symptoms can be caused by ingestion or skin exposure.

Caffeine

Caffeine is a natural stimulant found in coffee, chocolate, some teas, and energy drinks. Most people can tolerate up to about 400 milligrams of caffeine per day, but some individuals are very sensitive to caffeine. Sensitive individuals may experience rapid heartbeat, shakiness, anxiety, jitters, headaches, trouble sleeping, and/or upset stomach. These are nonallergic reactions to caffeine.

Recently, a few studies have documented individuals experiencing an anaphylactic response to caffeine, which may indicate that developing a caffeine allergy is possible. It is important to note that although caffeine allergies are very rare, an allergic response to caffeine needs to be treated as a medical emergency.

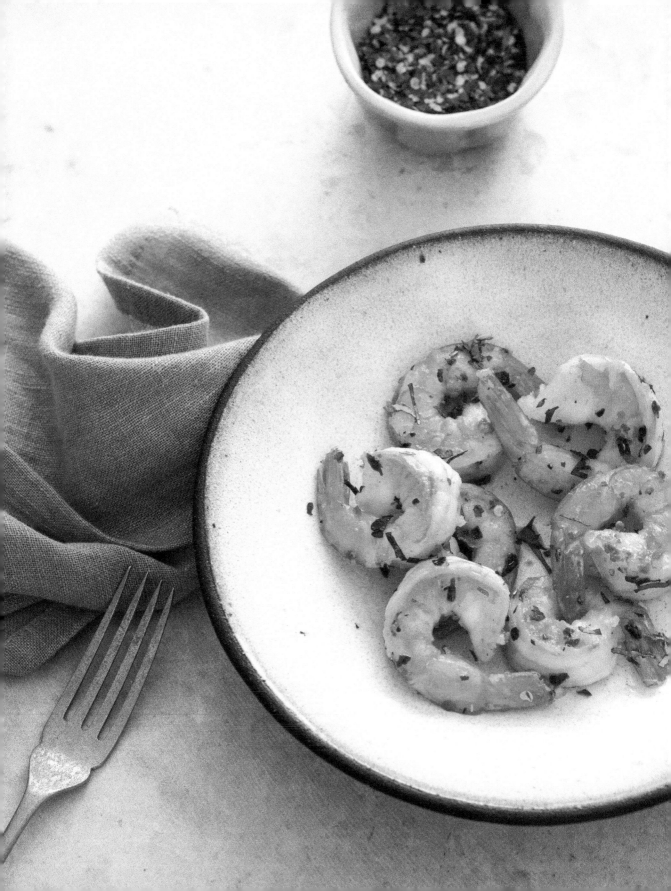

CHAPTER 3

Diagnosing Food Allergies and Sensitivities

Potential food allergies and intolerances should be evaluated and diagnosed by an allergist or other medical professional. This book is a tool to use with your health care provider to help pinpoint the cause of your symptoms. It is important not to self-diagnose, as you may miss the true cause of your symptoms and end up unnecessarily eliminating beneficial foods.

When meeting with your doctor or an allergist, the first step they will take is to obtain an accurate medical history. Completing the Elimination Diet outlined in this book can be a useful piece of your medical history that you share with your doctor in order to help reach an accurate diagnosis.

The Tests

Blood tests and skin prick tests can be an important part of a diagnosis, but they may not provide the most clear-cut answer for a food allergy or intolerance diagnosis. Moreover, results of blood tests and skin prick tests tend to be inconsistent, making them confusing when both are used on the same patient. Pair these tests with a detailed medical history, however, and your doctor will be able to help put the pieces of the puzzle together so that you can eat the foods that make you thrive.

BLOOD TESTS

The goal of blood tests is to detect antibodies present in the blood that are fighting against food allergens. The radioallergosorbent test (RAST) and fluorescent allergosorbent test (FAST) look for allergen-specific IgE. The enzyme-linked immunosorbent assay (ELISA) looks for allergen-specific IgE and IgG antibodies. To complete these tests, your doctor will draw a blood sample and send it to a lab where different foods can be tested.

It is important to note the degree of error in these tests. The body can make IgE antibodies for a component of a food, usually a protein, without actually causing a true food allergy, thereby creating a false positive result. Blood testing can be an effective part of the diagnosis plan for ruling out a food allergy, but changes to the diet do not need to be made if no symptoms are experienced when eating the potentially allergenic food.

SKIN PRICK TEST

To test for a food allergy, your allergist may suggest completing a skin prick test, which measures whether IgE antibodies are present for certain foods. These tests are fairly affordable, produce immediate results, and can be done in your doctor's office.

To complete the test, a drop of solution containing the potentially allergenic protein is placed on the skin. The skin is then pricked or scratched, allowing the allergen to enter the top layer of skin. The skin is then watched for a reaction. Similar to blood tests, skin prick tests can produce false positives.

Elimination Diet

An Elimination Diet temporarily removes specific foods from your diet for a certain period of time, then reintroduces those foods one at a time. Throughout the entire process, it's important to document the food you are consuming as well as any symptoms you may be experiencing, which is why I have included a sample journal for you beginning on page 49.

If you are experiencing symptoms from a food due to an allergy or intolerance, those symptoms should go away or decrease during the elimination period. If symptoms return when foods are added back into your diet, this is a strong indication you may have a food allergy or intolerance. At that point, it is important to meet with a doctor or allergist and share the notes in your journal so they can make an accurate diagnosis and help you come up with the next steps you should take.

If you already have a known food allergy, you should complete this Elimination Diet and reintroduction challenge under the supervision of a medical professional. Reintroducing a food you are allergic to may trigger a life-threatening allergic response, and your doctor may decide it is wisest to avoid it altogether.

The Elimination Diet takes place in two phases: an elimination phase and a reintroduction phase (also known as the challenge phase). Each phase lasts about two weeks. If your symptoms do not go away after completing the elimination phase, they may be caused by something other than a food allergy or intolerance, and it is best to talk with your doctor.

The reintroduction phase is the most important part of the diet. You will slowly bring foods back into your eating plan one by one, while documenting any symptoms or lack of symptoms. If you reintroduce a food and experience no symptoms, you do not have an allergy to or intolerance of that food and can continue consuming it regularly once the entire process is complete.

This Elimination Diet removes multiple foods at one time in an attempt to test for as many food allergies and sensitivities as possible, which is why it is important that you do not stay on this diet in the long term. Eliminating too many foods and food groups from your diet may cause nutritional deficiencies, which also have negative symptoms. The goal of this diet is to help you find the foods that allow you to feel your best, so you can reap the benefits of a balanced diet that includes as much variety as possible.

If you are experiencing symptoms such as skin rashes, hives, eczema, joint pain, headaches, fatigue, difficulty sleeping, difficulty or changes in breathing, bloating, stomach pain, runny eyes, stuffy nose, and/or changes in bowel movements, completing an Elimination Diet can help you determine if food is causing these symptoms. That being said, if you are not currently experiencing symptoms you feel may be related to the food you eat, there is no need to complete the Elimination Diet.

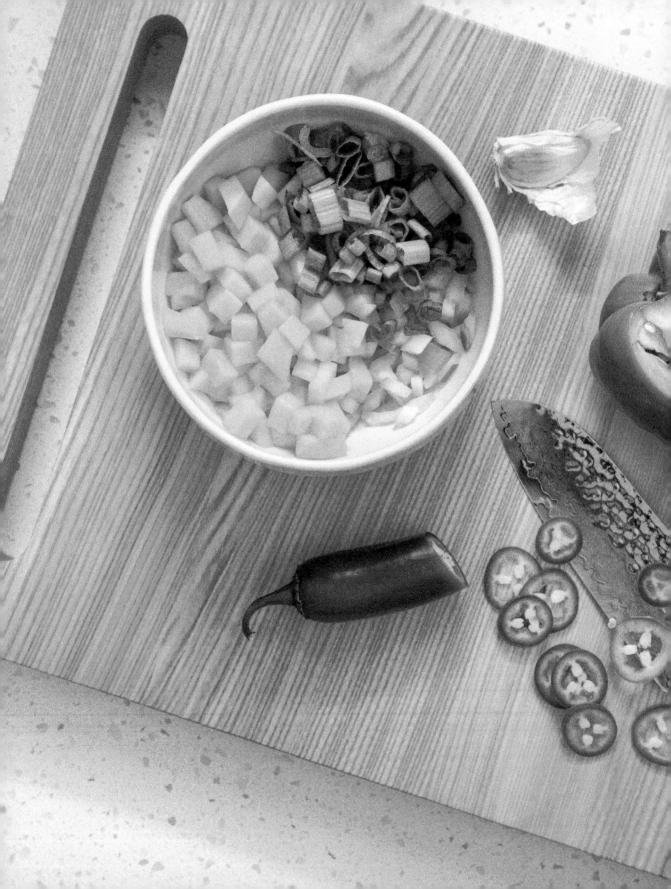

PART 2

The Elimination Diet

THE GOAL OF the Elimination Diet is to help you identify food allergies and intolerances. This can be a challenging task, so I have outlined how to go through this process, provided a meal plan for you to follow, and included a journal so you can take note of your symptoms throughout this journey. After you've become a food detective and figured out what may be causing your symptoms, you can share your experience and your journal with a health care professional to establish a diagnosis. Together, you can then come up with a plan so you can enjoy the widest variety of foods possible.

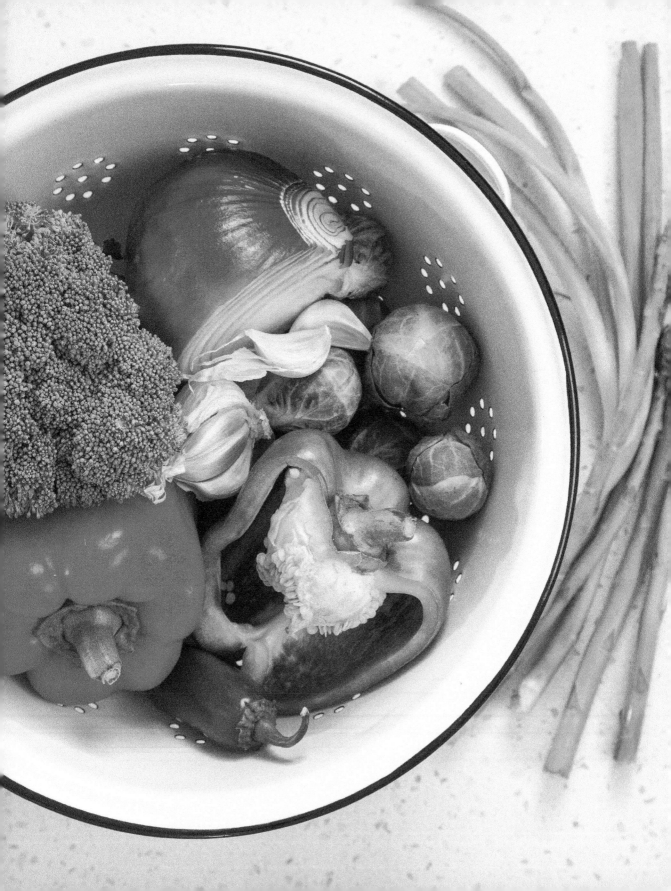

CHAPTER 4

The Elimination Phase

According to current research, completing an Elimination Diet followed by a reintroduction phase is necessary for the diagnosis of a food allergy or intolerance. Here, I outline the goal of the Elimination Diet, inform you of which foods you can eat during the 14-day elimination period and which foods you should avoid, offer tips for reading food labels, give you a meal plan (I promise you won't go hungry!), and provide a journal template for you to track symptoms.

The Goal

The goal of the Elimination Diet is to identify foods that cause reactions. While completing the elimination and challenge phases, it is important to document food and beverages consumed, along with any symptoms. This journal is a tool to use with a medical professional to create an eating plan that allows you to enjoy the widest variety of foods possible. The 14-day Elimination Diet plan focuses on the most common allergens, foods, and additives that are linked with food allergies and intolerances. These include milk/dairy, wheat, eggs, fish, shellfish, soy, peanuts, tree nuts, sesame, corn, gluten, lactose, nitrates and nitrites, histamines, MSG, sulfites, benzoates, artificial colors, and caffeine.

Because the Elimination Diet allows you to consume only a short list of foods during the elimination phase, this makes the step of reintroducing foods extremely important. Eating an overly restrictive diet for an extended period of time can lead to nutritional deficiencies, which have their own set of symptoms. Because of the limited food variety in this meal plan, I am not focusing on latex-fruit allergies, exercise-induced food allergies, or pollen-food allergies. If you suspect that one of these conditions matches your symptoms, it is important to work with a medical professional who specializes in allergies to confirm the diagnosis and create a plan that meets your specific needs.

Foods You Can Eat

These foods have a very low chance of triggering a reaction associated with a food allergy or intolerance. All of these foods are safe to consume during the elimination phase and are used in the recipes in part 3. It is important to focus on fresh foods during this Elimination Diet and limit the amount of packaged and commercially prepared foods you consume.

Fruit

- Apples
- Bananas
- Blueberries
- Dragon fruit
- Figs
- Guavas
- Kiwi
- Longans
- Lychees
- Mangos
- Melons
- Passion fruit
- Pears
- Pomegranates
- Rhubarb
- Star fruit

Vegetables

- Artichokes
- Asparagus
- Bell peppers
- Broccoli
- Brussels sprouts
- Cabbage
- Carrots
- Cauliflower
- Cucumbers
- Garlic
- Jalapeños and other hot peppers
- Kale
- Onions
- Parsnips
- Potatoes
- Rutabagas
- Scallions
- Squash, butternut and spaghetti
- Summer squash, including zucchini
- Sweet potatoes
- Turnips

Grains and Starches

- Buckwheat
- Oats (only certified gluten-free)
- Quinoa
- Rice (all kinds— brown rice, white rice, wild rice)
- Rice cakes, plain (only certified gluten-free)
- Rice noodles (only certified gluten-free)
- Soba noodles (only certified gluten-free)

Meat and Poultry

- Freeze-dried meat
- Plain, freshly cooked meat or poultry
- Previously cooked meat that is frozen immediately and reheated before consumption

Legumes

- Cannellini beans, canned
- Great northern beans, canned
- Peas
- Pinto beans, canned

Nuts and Seeds

- Chia seeds
- Flax seeds
- Hemp seeds
- Sunflower seeds and sunflower seed butter

Herbs/Seasonings

- Basil
- Cayenne pepper
- Chives
- Cumin
- Dill
- Oregano
- Paprika
- Sage

Fats and Oils

- Canola oil
- Homemade salad dressings (those included in this book)

Sugar and Sweeteners

- Agave syrup
- Brown rice syrup
- Cane sugar
- Maple syrup

Drinks

- Flax milk (check label for approved ingredients)
- Herbal tea
- Hemp milk (check label for approved ingredients)
- Oat milk (check label for approved ingredients and make sure oats are certified gluten-free)
- Rice milk (check label for approved ingredients)
- Water
- 100% apple juice
- 100% pomegranate juice

HERBAL TEAS FOR THE ELIMINATION PHASE

Many beverages contain ingredients that may trigger symptoms during the elimination phase. The best option is to drink water throughout the day, as hydration is important for everyone! For variety, here is a list of herbal teas that are suitable to enjoy during the elimination phase of the diet. Feel free to add one of the approved milks and a touch of sweetener from the list on page 30:

- Chamomile
- Echinacea
- Hibiscus
- Passionflower

- Peppermint
- Rooibos
- Rose hip
- Sage

Foods to Avoid

During the 14-Day Elimination Diet, you should avoid consuming the following foods, which may trigger a reaction due to a food intolerance or allergy. In the reintroduction phase, I will help you strategically add foods from each category back into your diet. As with the elimination phase, it will be important to journal your symptoms through the reintroduction phase with the template provided on page 50.

In addition to avoiding the foods listed on pages 32-39 during the elimination phase, it is important to focus on consuming fresh and minimally processed foods, drinking water as your main beverage, and staying away from caffeine and alcohol.

Milk/Dairy

- Baked goods
- Butter, butterfat, butter oil, butter acid, butter esters
- Buttermilk
- Caramel candies
- Cheese, or anything containing cheese
- Chocolate
- Cream (heavy, light, whipping)
- Curds
- Custard
- Gelato
- Ghee
- Half-and-half
- Ice cream
- Lunch meat, hot dogs, sausages (may contain casein or be sliced on the same machine as cheese)
- Margarine
- Milk in all forms (condensed, derivative, dry, evaporated, goat's milk, milk from other animals, low-fat, malted, milk fat, nonfat, powder, protein, skimmed, solids, whole)
- Nondairy products (they may contain casein—check the label)
- Nougat
- Pudding
- Shellfish (it is sometimes dipped in milk to reduce fishy odor)
- Some medications
- Some nondairy milks are manufactured in a facility with milk—check the label
- Sour cream, sour cream solids
- Sour milk solids
- Tuna (it sometimes contains casein)
- Yogurt

Wheat

- Bread
- Bread crumbs
- Cakes
- Candies
- Cereals
- Cracker crumbs
- Crackers
- Cookies
- Couscous
- Durum flour
- Farina
- Flour (particularly high-gluten or high-protein flour)
- Graham flour
- Lunch meat
- Muffins
- Pancakes
- Pasta
- Pies
- Sausages
- Semolina
- Snack foods
- Waffles
- Wheat bran
- Wheat germ

Egg

- Baked goods
- Egg in all forms (dried, powdered, solids, white, yolk)
- Egg substitutes
- Eggnog
- Foam on alcoholic drinks or specialty coffees
- Ice cream (check the label)
- Marshmallows
- Marzipan
- Mayonnaise
- Meringue (meringue powder)
- Nougat
- Pastas
- Pretzels (check the label)
- Processed meat, meat loaf, meatballs
- Puddings and custards
- Salad dressings
- Some medications
- Some vaccines
- Specialty coffee drinks and bars (check the label)
- Surimi
- Traditional wheat pasta

Fish

- All types of fish (fresh, canned, smoked, or frozen)
- Barbecue sauce (check the ingredient label for Worcestershire sauce)
- Caesar dressing (may contain anchovies)
- Fish oil
- Imitation or artificial fish
- Wine and beer made with isinglass
- Worcestershire sauce (may contain anchovies)

Shellfish

- Clams
- Crab
- Crawfish
- Lobster
- Mussels
- Octopus
- Oysters
- Scallops
- Shrimp/prawns
- Snails
- Squid

Soy

- Bean curd
- Edamame
- Miso
- Natto
- Shoyu
- Soy in all forms (soy cheese, soy fiber, soy flour, soy grits, soy ice cream, soy milk, soy nuts, soy sprouts, soy yogurt)
- Soy-based cooking sprays
- Soy-based margarines
- Soy oil
- Soy sauce
- Soya
- Soybeans (curd, granules)
- Tamari
- Tempeh
- Textured vegetable protein (TVP)
- Tofu
- Unlabeled breads and baked goods

Peanuts

- Artificial nuts
- Baked goods such as cookies or pastries (if you don't know the ingredients)
- Beer nuts
- Candy (check the label)
- Cereals and granola (check the label)
- Ice cream, frozen desserts
- Marzipan (usually made with almonds but sometimes with peanuts—check the label)
- Mixed nuts
- Nougat
- Nut butter (check the label)
- Nut meats
- Nut pieces
- Peanut butter
- Peanut flour
- Peanut oil
- Peanuts
- Pet food (the worry isn't that you'll eat it, but if you have a serious allergy, skin contact with it could provoke a reaction)
- Salad dressing (check the label)
- Whole-grain bread (check the label)

Tree Nuts

- Almonds
- Brazil nuts
- Cashews
- Chestnuts
- Coconut
- Hazelnuts/filberts
- Hickory nuts
- Macadamia nuts
- Mixed nuts
- Nuts and nut products
- Pecans
- Pistachios
- Walnuts

Sesame

- Falafel
- Flavor blends or spice/ herb blends (check the label)
- Flavored rice noodles, kebab, stir-fries
- Gingelly, gingelly oil
- Gomasio (sesame salt)
- Gomadofu (Japanese dessert)
- Halvah
- Herbs and herbal drinks
- Margarine
- Pasteli (Greek dessert)
- Processed meats and sausages
- Protein and energy bars
- Sesame flour
- Sesame oil
- Sesame paste
- Sesame salt
- Sesame seeds
- Sushi
- Tahini, tahina, tehina
- Tempeh
- Turkish cake
- Vegetarian burgers
- Read the ingredient labels for Asian and Middle Eastern packaged foods, sauces, condiments, cereal, baked goods, snack foods, dips, herbal drinks, processed meats and sausages, soups, cosmetics, medications, and supplements

Corn

- Baking powder
- Caramel
- Corn (canned, fresh, frozen, niblets, on the cob)
- Corn flour
- Corn oil
- Corn sugar
- Corn sweetener
- Corn syrup (including high-fructose corn syrup)
- Cornflakes
- Cornmeal
- Cornstarch
- Creamed corn
- Grits
- Hominy
- Maize
- Malt
- Mixed vegetables (check the label)
- Polenta
- Popcorn
- Semolina
- Textured vegetable protein (TVP)
- Read the ingredient labels for Mexican packaged foods, cereal, baked goods, snack foods, syrups, canned fruits, beverages, jams, jellies, cookies, lunch meats, candies, convenience food, vanilla extract, and medications

Gluten

- Barley
- Brewer's yeast
- Malt
- Oats (if not certified gluten-free)
- Rye
- Triticale
- Wheat

Lactose

- This sugar is found in many dairy products, unless reduced through the fermentation process; most dairy products should be avoided.

Nitrates and Nitrites

- Alcohol
- Arugula/rocket
- Beets and beet greens
- Canned meat
- Celery
- Cured and/or smoked meats and fish (salami, hot dogs, pepperoni, bacon, ham, processed meat)
- Fennel
- Frozen pizza
- Green beans
- Kohlrabi
- Leeks
- Lettuce
- Lunch meat
- Parsley
- Processed cheese
- Radishes
- Spinach
- Strawberries
- Turnip greens

Histamines

- Alcohol
- Anise
- Apricots
- Avocados
- Bleached flour
- Buttermilk
- Canned meat or fish
- Cheese made by fermentation
- Cherries
- Chili powder
- Chocolate
- Cinnamon
- Cloves
- Cola-type carbonated beverages
- Commercial candies
- Commercial frosting
- Commercial sweeteners
- Commercially prepared desserts
- Cottage cheese

- Cranberries
- Crème fraîche
- Currants
- Curry powder
- Dates
- Dried fruit
- Egg whites
- Eggplant
- Fats or oils with added color or preservatives
- Fermented drinks (kombucha, kefir)
- Fermented foods (sauerkraut, kimchi)
- Flavored coffee
- Flavored drinks
- Flavored milk
- Foods labeled with "spices"
- Garbanzo beans/chickpeas
- Grapefruit
- Grapes
- Gravy from mixes or cans
- Leftover cooked meat
- Lemons
- Lentils
- Limes
- Loganberries
- Margarine
- Mulberries
- Nectarines
- Nonalcoholic beer and wine
- Nut and seed mixtures with artificial flavoring
- Nutmeg
- Olives and olive oil
- Oranges
- Papayas
- Pineapple
- Plums
- Prepackaged food
- Processed cheese products
- Processed, smoked, pickled, and/or fermented meats like lunch meat, sausage, wieners, hot dogs, bologna, salami, pepperoni, bacon, ham
- Prunes
- Pumpkin and pumpkin seeds
- Raisins
- Raspberries
- Red beans (kidney and adzuki beans)
- Ricotta cheese
- Ripe tomatoes (green tomatoes are fine)
- Saskatoon berries
- Seasoning packets and mixtures
- Sour cream
- Soy products (miso, soy lecithin, soy milk, soy sauce, tofu, tempeh)
- Soybeans
- Spinach
- Strawberries
- Tea (black and green)
- Thyme
- Vinegar
- Yogurt

Monosodium Glutamate (MSG)

- Accent seasoning
- Bottled and canned sauces
- Canned meat
- Canned soups and dry soup mixes
- Cookies and crackers
- Croutons
- Cured meats
- Diet foods
- Freeze-dried foods
- Frozen foods
- Gravy mixes
- Potato chips
- Prepared dinners and side dishes
- Prepared salads, salad dressings, mayonnaise
- Prepared snacks
- Spice and seasoning blends

Sulfites

- Beer
- Canned crab meat
- Canned fruit
- Canned vegetables
- Caramel
- Cider
- Cider vinegar
- Dehydrated fruit
- Dehydrated mashed potatoes
- Dehydrated vegetables
- Desiccated coconut
- Dried fruit
- Fermented vegetables
- Flavorings
- Frozen mushrooms
- Fruit-based milk and cream desserts
- Fruit fillings
- Fruit juices
- Fruit spread
- Garlic powder
- Gelatin
- Ground ginger
- Jams and jellies
- Ketchup
- Maraschino cherries
- Pickled onions
- Pickled red cabbage
- Preserved egg yolk
- Quick-frozen French fries
- Quick-frozen shrimp and lobster
- Relish
- Sausage
- Soft drinks
- Soup packets
- Tomato paste
- Vegetable juice
- Wine

Caffeine

- Chocolate
- Chocolate-flavored food
- Coffee, regular and decaf
- Energy drinks
- Soda
- Tea (green, black, red, and white)

Benzoates

- Apricots
- Avocados
- Barbecue sauce
- Canned beets
- Canned red beans
- Caviar
- Cheesecake mix
- Cherries
- Cinnamon
- Cloves
- Cod
- Cranberries
- Dessert sauces
- Flavored coffee
- Flavored syrups
- Fruit juice and fruit juice concentrates
- Fruit pies
- Grapefruit
- Honey
- Jam
- Margarine
- Marinated fish
- Nectarines
- Nutmeg
- Olives
- Oranges
- Papayas
- Peaches
- Pickles
- Pimentos
- Plums
- Prawns
- Prunes
- Pumpkin
- Raspberries
- Salad dressing
- Soft drinks
- Soy sauce
- Soybeans
- Spinach
- Strawberries
- Taco sauce
- Tea (black and green)
- Thyme
- Yogurt

Artificial Colors

- Bottled sauces
- Cake mix
- Candies
- Canned applesauce
- Canned pears
- Canned pie fillings
- Canned shrimp/prawns
- Chewing gum
- Commercial salad dressings
- Fruit punch
- Gelatin dessert mix
- Gravy mixes
- Ice cream
- Instant pudding
- Jams and jellies
- Liquid vitamin C
- Mustard
- Packaged convenience food
- Pickles
- Sherbet
- Smoked fish
- Soup, dried and canned
- Yogurt

LEARNING THE SECRET LANGUAGE OF FOOD LABELS

Make sure to check the ingredient label! Some of these ingredients may seem unfamiliar to you, but they are just different names for the foods or additives that may be causing you discomfort. At first, it may take a little extra time at the store as you get used to looking at the ingredient list, but fortunately, the Food Allergen Labeling and Consumer Protection Act (FALCPA) of 2004 made things a bit easier for those with food allergies and intolerances. FALCPA requires that foods containing one or more of the eight major food allergens (milk, wheat, eggs, fish, shellfish, soy, peanuts, tree nuts) must be labeled to make it easy to identify the allergen.

Milk

- Butter flavor
- Casein
- Casein hydrolysate
- Caseinates (in all forms)
- Cheese flavor
- Diacetyl
- Hydrolysates
- Lactalbumin, lactalbumin phosphate
- Lactoferrin
- Lactose (or anything with the prefix "lact")
- Lactulose
- Milk protein hydrolysate
- Nisin
- Recaldent
- Rennet casein
- Tagatose
- Whey (in all forms)
- Whey protein hydrolysate

Wheat

- Gelatinized starch
- Gluten
- High-gluten flour
- High-protein flour
- Modified starch
- Vegetable gum
- Vegetable starch
- Vital gluten
- Wheat gluten

Corn

- Cellulose
- Citric acid
- Corn alcohol
- Dextrate
- Dextrin
- Dextrose
- Glucose
- Inositol
- Maltodextrin
- Maltodextrose
- Modified starch
- Monosodium glutamate
- Sodium erythorbate
- Sorbitol
- Starch
- Vegetable gum

Egg

- Albumin (albumen)
- Lecithin
- Lysozyme
- Ovalbumin

Peanuts

- Arachis
- Goobers
- Ground nuts
- Lupin (or lupine)
- Mandelonas
- Monkey nuts
- Peanut protein hydrolysate

Sesame

- Benne, benne seed, benniseed
- Gingelly, gingelly oil
- Sesamol
- Sesamum indicum
- Sesemolina
- Sim sim
- Til
- Vegetable paste
- Vegetable protein
- Vegetable starch
- Xanthan gum

Histamines

- Hydrolyzed lecithin

Nitrates/Nitrites

- Potassium nitrate
- Potassium nitrite
- Sodium nitrate
- Sodium nitrite

MSG

- Ajinomoto
- Chinese seasoning
- Glutacyl
- Glutavene
- Hydrolyzed plant protein (HPP)
- Hydrolyzed [plant source name] protein (e.g., hydrolyzed soy protein)
- Hydrolyzed vegetable protein (HVP)
- Flavorings
- Gourmet powder
- Kombu extract
- Mei-jing
- Natural flavoring (may be HVP)
- RL-50
- Subu
- Vetsin
- Wei-jing
- Zest

Soy

- Hydrolyzed plant protein (HPP)
- Lecithin

Sulfites

- Potassium bisulfite
- Potassium metabisulfite
- Sodium bisulfite
- Sodium dithionite
- Sodium metabisulfite
- Sodium sulfite
- Sulfur dioxide
- Sulfurous acid

- FD&C Blue #1, Brilliant Blue
- FD&C Blue #2, Indigotine
- FD&C Green #3, Fast Green
- FD&C Citrus Red #2, Citrus Red #2
- FD&C Red #3, Erythrosine

- FD&C Red #40, Allura Red
- FD&C Yellow #5, Tartrazine
- FD&C Yellow #6, Sunset Yellow
- Orange B

The Meal Plan

This meal plan gives suggestions for breakfast, lunch, dinner, and a snack utilizing recipes from this book and foods that are on the Foods You Can Eat list (pages 28–31). This is a sample meal plan to make the Elimination Diet as simple for you as possible, but please feel free to mix and match with recipes included in this book. They all taste delicious, and I want this to be a flavorful and satisfying time of eating for you as you work as a detective to figure out what is causing your symptoms. If you feel hungry between meals or in the evening, please feel free to enjoy more food. If you feel overly full or unable to finish the portion recommended, I suggest you listen to your hunger and fullness cues and stop eating when you feel full and satisfied.

14-Day Elimination Diet Meal Plan

DAY #	1	2	3	4	5	6	7
BREAKFAST	Overnight Steel-Cut Oatmeal (page 60) with pear and sunflower seed butter	Chia Pudding Power Bowl (page 62)	Overnight Steel-Cut Oatmeal (page 60) with kiwi and hemp seeds	Tropical Green Smoothie (page 65)	Overnight Steel-Cut Oatmeal (page 60) with blueberries, banana, and chia seeds	Buckwheat-Banana Pancakes (page 63)	Banana Oatmeal with Hemp and Chia Seeds (page 61) with banana and sunflower seed butter
LUNCH	Superfood Salad (page 73) and Oatmeal Snack Bite (page 167)	Mediterranean Mason Jar Pesto Salad (page 78) with Super-Seedy Crackers (page 173) and Garlic-Dill White Bean Dip (page 174)	Superfood Salad (page 73) and Oatmeal Snack Bite (page 167)	Mediterranean Mason Jar Pesto Salad (page 78) with Super-Seedy Crackers (page 173) and Garlic-Dill White Bean Dip (page 174)	Mediterranean Mason Jar Pesto Salad (page 78) with Super-Seedy Crackers (page 173) and Garlic-Dill White Bean Dip (page 174)	Mediterranean Mason Jar Pesto Salad (page 78) with Super-Seedy Crackers (page 173) and a pear	Soba Noodle Bowl with Chicken and Sunflower Sauce (page 92)
DINNER	Back Pocket Stir-Fry with Rice Noodles (page 123)	Sweet Potato Sunflower Soup (page 100)	Italian Chicken Burgers with Roasted Vegetables (page 127) and Garlic-Roasted Broccoli (page 154)	Roasted Turmeric Chicken with Broccoli (page 111)	Sweet Potato Sunflower Soup (page 100)	Beef and Broccoli Bowl (page 132)	Slow Cooker Maple-Garlic Chicken (page 109) with Garlic-Ginger Bok Choy (page 159) and Simple Brown Rice (page 162)
SNACK	Fresh blueberries and sliced banana	Pear and sunflower seed butter	Mango-Banana Nice Cream (page 166)	Blueberry Bread (page 171)	Mango-Banana Nice Cream (page 166)	Blueberry Bread (page 171)	Sliced carrots and cucumbers

8	9	10	11	12	13	14
Blueberry Breakfast Smoothie (page 64)	Overnight Steel-Cut Oatmeal (page 60) with pear and sunflower seed butter	Banana Oatmeal with Hemp and Chia Seeds (page 61) with blueberries	Overnight Steel-Cut Oatmeal (page 60) with blueberries, banana, and chia seeds	Tropical Green Smoothie (page 65)	Overnight Steel-Cut Oatmeal (page 60) with kiwi and hemp seeds	Chia Pudding Power Bowl (page 62)
Kitchen Sink Salad (page 70) and Banana-Apple Buckwheat Muffin (page 170)	Sweet Potato Buddha Bowl (page 82) with sliced banana and blueberries	Kitchen Sink Salad (page 70) and Banana-Apple Buckwheat Muffin (page 170)	Bell Pepper and Basil Wild Rice Bowl (page 86) with pear and sunflower seed butter	Sweet Potato Buddha Bowl (page 82) and Banana-Apple Buckwheat Muffin (page 170)	Bell Pepper and Basil Wild Rice Bowl (page 86) and Oatmeal Snack Bite (page 167)	Sweet Potato Falafel Bowl (page 84) and Oatmeal Snack Bite (page 167)
White Bean Turkey Chili (page 104)	Slow Cooker Maple-Garlic Chicken (page 109) with Simple Brown Rice (page 162) and Simple Roasted Vegetables (page 156)	White Bean Turkey Chili (page 104)	Chicken Skewers with Basil Pesto (page 121) with Roasted Turnips with Kale and White Beans (page 153)	Chicken Soup with Quinoa and Greens (page 97)	Sweet Potato Zoodle Soup with Creamy Turmeric Sauce (page 102)	Mango Chicken (page 120) with Garlic-Roasted Broccoli (page 154)
Blueberry Bread (page 171)	Creamy Mango Lassi (page 172)	Blueberry Bread (page 171)	Chopped carrots and cucumbers	Pear and sunflower seed butter	Mango Oat Crumble Bar (page 168)	Mango Oat Crumble Bar (page 168)

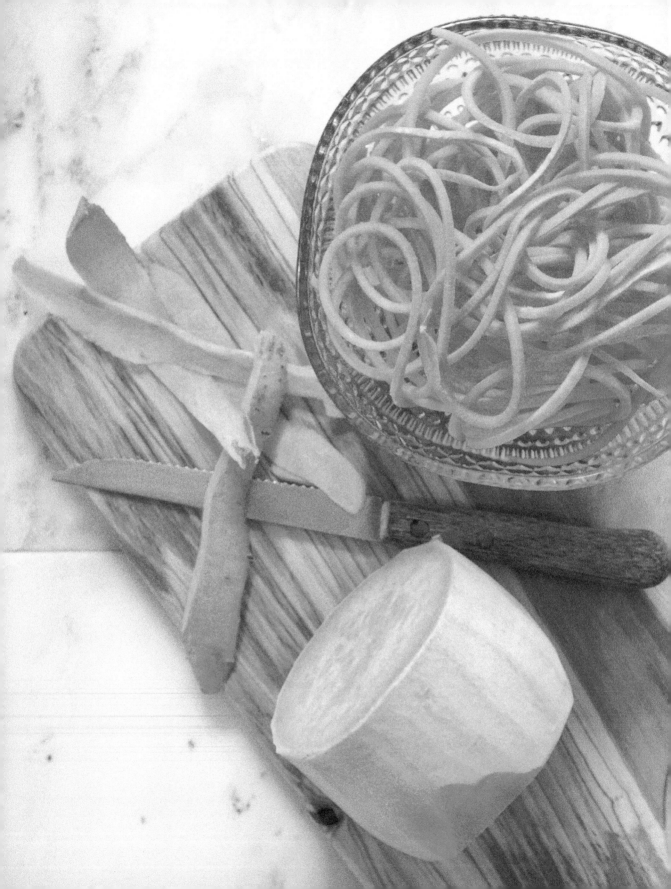

CHAPTER 5

The Reintroduction Phase

After following the Elimination Diet for two weeks, the next step in identifying foods and food additives that may be causing an allergy or intolerance is to reintroduce items from each category individually so that you can clearly identify when symptoms are present and what may be causing them.

Easy Does It: One at a Time

To reintroduce foods that have been eliminated during the initial two-week period, it is important to consume something from each category one at a time. Many reactions to foods and food additives are not severe, and a food challenge can be safely completed at home.

Because unnecessary food restriction can have negative health and emotional effects, adding foods back into your diet may be the most important part of the Elimination Diet. By challenging the different categories of food and reintroducing foods into your diet one by one, you will be able to include a wider variety of safe, nutritious foods that allow you to feel your best.

Please note that for any foods that have previously caused an anaphylactic reaction or could cause an anaphylactic reaction or could cause a severe asthmatic reaction, the reintroduction should occur under medical supervision in a well-equipped medical facility.

Important steps to follow when reintroducing foods:

- Continue to eat foods allowed on the Elimination Diet (pages 28–31). The only change is adding a food from a specific category during each challenge.

- Complete a screening challenge so you can have a measure of safety prior to consuming the foods (this is especially important if working with a child).

   - Place food on the skin of your cheek (outside your mouth) and observe for a reaction in that area. Symptoms include reddening, blistering, or irritation.

   - If you don't witness a symptom and experience no reaction, move on to a lip food challenge by placing the food on the outer border of the lower lip for two minutes, then watch the place where you placed the food for 30 minutes. Symptoms include swelling, reddening, irritation where the food was placed, rash on the cheek or chin, stuffy nose, or red/watery eyes.

- If placing the food on the lip causes no reaction, consume each food three times on each test day at four-hour intervals in increasing doses, carefully monitoring your symptoms or lack of symptoms. I have structured this to incorporate the foods at breakfast, lunch, and dinner.

- If you encounter symptoms, they should be the same ones you experienced prior to completing the 14-day Elimination Diet. Any new symptom is unlikely due to the food and should be mentioned to a medical care provider. You should try reintroducing the food that may be causing new symptoms again after two weeks.

- **If symptoms develop at any time during the reintroduction, stop consumption of that food immediately.** You should continue to follow the Elimination Diet until all symptoms are gone. You can resume testing the next category 48 hours (two days) after the symptoms have gone away.

- If you don't experience symptoms on Day 1 of introducing a food/category, Day 2 is a monitoring day for delayed reactions. On Day 2, you will consume the foods allowed in the Elimination Diet but none of the food you are testing.

- If you don't have any symptoms on Day 1 or 2, the food can be labeled as safe. On Day 3, introduce the next category of food. You will continue to follow the Elimination Diet until all categories of foods and additives are reintroduced one at a time. After all testing is completed, you can freely eat the foods that did not cause any reaction.

- Sometimes on Day 1 or 2, you may experience symptoms that are so mild you will be uncertain whether they're related to the food you're reintroducing or to another event entirely. If this happens, on Day 3 you will consume the same food as you did on Day 1 in larger portions and in three increasing doses. Day 4 is another monitoring day. If the test food is causing the reaction, symptoms will increase in severity. If the food is not responsible for the reactions, the symptoms will go away or stay the same.

- You can reintroduce foods in any order you like, as long as this is done one category at a time.

Keep a Journal

This is your chance to act as a detective and figure out what is causing your symptoms. By completing a daily food journal, you will hopefully notice a correlation between some of your symptoms and foods that you are or are not eating. Once you have completed the entire challenge phase, this will be an excellent tool to take with you to a doctor or allergist so they can make an accurate diagnosis and help you come up with a plan.

Day 1 (*Italicized words are examples of what you might write in.*)

MEAL	FOOD/DRINK/SUPPLEMENTS	SYMPTOMS	CHANGES
BREAKFAST 8 A.M. REINTRODUCTION DAY 1: WHEAT	*-Overnight Steel-Cut Oatmeal made with certified gluten-free oats, rice milk, salt, and about 1 tablespoon sunflower seed butter. Added 1 tablespoon wheat germ.* *-Now Probiotic-10, 25 billion* *-16 oz. water*	*Started to feel headache coming on.*	*Never had headaches when consuming wheat before the Elimination Diet, so this symptom is probably unrelated.*
LUNCH 12 P.M.	*Superfood Salad and Oatmeal Snack Bite with 1 slice sourdough bread (ingredients are wheat, water, and salt)*		
SNACK 3 P.M.			
DINNER 6 P.M.	*Back Pocket Stir-Fry with wheat spaghetti instead of rice noodles*		

What to Do If You Have a Reaction

If you have a reaction or notice symptoms develop at any time during the reintroduction phase, it is important to stop consuming that food immediately. Continue to eat foods on the Foods You Can Eat list (pages 28–31), use the recipes in this book, and make sure to complete the journal explaining what you experienced. You can continue testing other foods 48 hours after your symptoms are gone.

KNOW THE SIGNS

You will experience symptoms you have experienced in the past. Each person is individual in how they respond to potentially triggering foods.

- Anaphylaxis
- Asthma-like symptoms
- Bloating or abdominal pain
- Blurry vision
- Diarrhea, loose stools
- Dizziness
- Facial numbness
- Gas
- Hives
- Migraine or headache
- Nausea/vomiting
- Skin rash
- Skin reddening or itching
- Stuffy nose
- Swelling
- Throat tightening
- Tight chest
- Tingling fingers and feet
- Watery and red eyes

Reintroduction Schedule

When introducing foods back into the Elimination Diet, you can introduce foods in the order that you prefer. It is important to maintain your journal throughout the entire process and continue eating the foods listed on pages 28–31 in the Elimination Diet. This will make it easier to identify which foods are causing you to have a reaction. Please refer to the steps on pages 48–49 to know what to do when reintroducing a food.

REINTRODUCTION	WHEN/HOW TO ADD THE TEST FOOD IN
WHEAT/GLUTEN	**Breakfast:** Mix 1 tablespoon wheat germ into Overnight Steel-Cut Oatmeal (page 60), Banana Oatmeal with Hemp and Chia Seeds (page 61), Tropical Green Smoothie (page 65), or Blueberry Breakfast Smoothie (page 64). **Lunch:** Have a slice of sourdough bread (ingredients should be only flour, water, and salt) along with one of the bowls or salads in chapter 7. **Dinner:** Use traditional wheat pasta in place of the spaghetti squash in Spaghetti Squash and Meatballs (page 136), the soba noodles in Soba Noodle Bowl with Chicken and Sunflower Sauce (page 92), or the rice noodles in Back Pocket Stir-Fry with Rice Noodles (page 123).
MILK/DAIRY	**Breakfast:** Add ¼ cup plain, unsweetened yogurt to Banana Oatmeal with Hemp and Chia Seeds (page 61), Chia Pudding Power Bowl (page 62), Tropical Green Smoothie (page 65), or Blueberry Breakfast Smoothie (page 64). **Lunch:** Add ¼ cup grated or crumbled cheese to Meal Prep Quinoa Taco Bowl (page 89; use cheddar), Kitchen Sink Salad (page 70; use feta), or Mediterranean Mason Jar Pesto Salad (page 78; use Parmesan). **Dinner:** Serve Italian Chicken Burgers (page 127) with 1 to 2 cheese slices per burger or sprinkle ¼ cup grated Parmesan onto a serving of Chicken Skewers with Basil Pesto (page 121) with Roasted Turnips with Kale and White Beans (page 153).
EGG	**Breakfast:** Make Banana-Apple Buckwheat Muffins (page 170) with 2 eggs instead of 2 flax eggs and eat one muffin for breakfast with a pear or a side of blueberries. **Lunch:** Add ½ hard-boiled egg to a serving of Bell Pepper and Basil Wild Rice Bowl (page 86), Sweet Potato Buddha Bowl (page 82), or Superfood Salad (page 73). **Dinner:** Eat 1 hard-boiled egg with your dinner.
FISH	**Breakfast:** Eat 2 tablespoons canned tuna with breakfast. **Lunch:** Add ¼ cup canned tuna to a serving of Roasted Cauliflower Quinoa Bowl (page 87), Spring Roll Bowl (page 90), or Mediterranean Mason Jar Pesto Salad (page 78). **Dinner:** Add ⅓ cup canned tuna to a serving of Sweet Potato Buddha Bowl (page 82), Roasted Vegetable and Brown Rice Bowl with Green Sauce (page 80), or Herby Cauliflower Salad (page 75).
SHELLFISH	**Breakfast**: Eat 2 cooked shrimp with breakfast. **Lunch:** Add 2 ounces cooked shrimp to a serving of Bell Pepper and Basil Wild Rice Bowl (page 86), Spring Roll Bowl (page 90), or Golden Roasted Cauliflower and Brown Rice Salad (page 68). **Dinner:** Replace meat or chicken with 4 ounces cooked shrimp in a serving of Soba Noodle Bowl with Chicken and Sunflower Sauce (page 92), Spaghetti Squash and Meatballs (page 136), or Back Pocket Stir-Fry with Rice Noodles (page 123).

REINTRODUCTION	WHEN/HOW TO ADD THE TEST FOOD IN
SOY	**Breakfast**: Add 2 tablespoons drained tofu to Tropical Green Smoothie (page 65) or Blueberry Breakfast Smoothie (page 64). **Lunch:** Add ¼ cup roasted tofu cubes to a serving of Kitchen Sink Salad (page 70), Roasted Cauliflower Quinoa Bowl (page 87), or Roasted Vegetable and Brown Rice Bowl with Green Sauce (page 80). **Dinner:** Add ½ cup roasted tofu cubes to a serving of Spring Roll Bowl (page 90) or Roasted Cauliflower Quinoa Bowl (page 87), or in place of the chicken in Soba Noodle Bowl with Chicken and Sunflower Sauce (page 92).
PEANUTS	**Breakfast**: Add 1 teaspoon peanut butter to Overnight Steel-Cut Oatmeal (page 60) or Banana Oatmeal with Hemp and Chia Seeds (page 61), or in place of the sunflower seed butter in Chia Pudding Power Bowl (page 62). **Lunch:** Use 1 tablespoon peanut butter instead of the sunflower butter in Slow Cooker Pork Stir-Fry (page 146), Kitchen Sink Salad (page 70), or Soba Noodle Bowl with Chicken and Sunflower Sauce (page 92). **Dinner:** Serve 2 tablespoons peanut butter with pear or banana on the side of dinner.
TREE NUTS	**Breakfast**: Sprinkle 1 tablespoon roughly chopped cashews or almonds on Overnight Steel-Cut Oatmeal (page 60), Banana Oatmeal with Hemp and Chia Seeds (page 61), or Chia Pudding Power Bowl (page 62). **Lunch:** Sprinkle 2 tablespoons roughly chopped cashews or almonds over Bell Pepper and Basil Wild Rice Bowl (page 86), Sweet Potato Falafel Bowl (page 84), or Sweet Potato Buddha Bowl (page 82). **Dinner:** Sprinkle 3 tablespoons roughly chopped cashews over a side of Garlic-Ginger Bok Choy (page 159) or Garlic-Roasted Broccoli (page 154), or on Beef and Broccoli Bowl (page 132).
SESAME	**Breakfast**: Add 1 tablespoon sesame seeds to Overnight Steel-Cut Oatmeal (page 60), Banana Oatmeal with Hemp and Chia Seeds (page 61), Chia Pudding Power Bowl (page 62), Tropical Green Smoothie (page 65), or Blueberry Breakfast Smoothie (page 64). **Lunch:** Add 2 tablespoons sesame seeds to Sweet Potato Buddha Bowl (page 82), Roasted Cauliflower Quinoa Bowl (page 87), Superfood Salad (page 73), or Spring Roll Bowl (page 90). **Dinner:** Add 3 tablespoons sesame seeds to a serving of Butternut Squash and White Bean Soup (page 101), White Bean Turkey Chili (page 104), or Sheet Pan Chicken Breasts with Garlicky Greens (page 112).

REINTRODUCTION	WHEN/HOW TO ADD THE TEST FOOD IN
CORN	**Breakfast:** Eat 1 tablespoon drained and rinsed canned corn with breakfast. **Lunch:** Add ¼ cup drained and rinsed canned corn to Meal Prep Quinoa Taco Bowl (page 89), Roasted Vegetable and Brown Rice Bowl with Green Sauce (page 80), or Mediterranean Mason Jar Pesto Salad (page 78). **Dinner:** Add ½ cup drained and rinsed canned corn to White Bean Turkey Chili (page 104) or Back Pocket Stir-Fry with Rice Noodles (page 123), or alongside Paprika Drumsticks (page 125).
LACTOSE	**Breakfast:** Add ½ cup dairy milk to Overnight Steel-Cut Oatmeal (page 60) or replace ½ cup of the nondairy milk with ½ cup dairy milk in either Blueberry Breakfast Smoothie (page 64) or Tropical Green Smoothie (page 65). **Lunch:** Drink 1 cup dairy milk with lunch or mix into Mango-Banana Nice Cream (page 166). **Dinner:** Drink 1¼ cups dairy milk with dinner or mix into Creamy Mango Lassi (page 172).
NITRATES AND NITRITES Note: To be sure the lunch meat turkey has nitrates or nitrites, check the ingredient label for sodium nitrate, potassium nitrate, sodium nitrite, or potassium nitrate. You can ask the individual working at the deli counter to help you.	**Breakfast**: Add 1 slice lunch meat turkey that contains nitrates or nitrites to your normal breakfast from one of the recipes in this book. **Lunch:** Add 2 slices lunch meat turkey that includes nitrates or nitrites to a serving of Bell Pepper and Basil Wild Rice Bowl (page 86), Roasted Vegetable and Brown Rice Bowl with Green Sauce (page 80), or Superfood Salad (page 73). **Dinner:** Add 3 slices lunch meat turkey that includes nitrates or nitrites to a serving of Roasted Brussels Sprouts with Wild Rice (page 157), Dilled Bean Salad with Carrots and Quinoa (page 152), Mediterranean Roasted Asparagus (page 155), or Perfectly Cooked Quinoa (page 163).
HISTAMINES Note: Histamine intolerance is hard to test for with a food challenge because there may be overlap in foods consumed (for example, the cheese and yogurt tested in dairy and the lunch meat used in nitrates/nitrites are higher in histamines).	**Breakfast**: Add ½ cup strawberries to Overnight Steel-Cut Oatmeal (page 60), use as a topping for Banana Oatmeal with Hemp and Chia Seeds (page 61), or mix into Buckwheat-Banana Pancakes (page 63). **Lunch:** Enjoy ½ cup strawberries with your lunch and add ¼ cup cherry tomatoes to Sunflower and White Bean Salad (page 72), Bell Pepper and Basil Wild Rice Bowl (page 86), or Spring Roll Bowl (page 90). **Dinner:** Enjoy ½ cup strawberries with dinner and add ½ cup cherry tomatoes to Sheet Pan Chicken Breasts with Garlicky Greens (page 112), Taco Stuffed Sweet Potatoes (page 140), or Chicken Skewers with Basil Pesto (page 121).

REINTRODUCTION	WHEN/HOW TO ADD THE TEST FOOD IN
MSG Note: Many grocery stores sell MSG (such as Accent brand seasoning); add a little bit to each meal. Each meal should be made from foods allowed during the Elimination Diet or a recipe from this book.	**Breakfast:** Sprinkle a small dash into your morning meal. **Lunch:** Sprinkle 2 small dashes into your meal. **Dinner:** Sprinkle ⅛ teaspoon into your meal.
SULFITES Note: Purchase regular dried mango with sulfur dioxide as an ingredient.	**Breakfast:** Add ½ ounce dried mango as a topping to Banana Oatmeal with Hemp and Chia Seeds (page 61), Overnight Steel-Cut Oatmeal (page 60) or Chia Pudding Power Bowl (page 62). **Lunch:** Eat 1 ounce dried mango with lunch. **Dinner:** Eat 1½ ounces dried mango with dinner.
BENZOATES Note: Cinnamon has a high amount of naturally occurring benzoate.	**Breakfast:** Add ⅛ teaspoon ground cinnamon to a serving of Banana Oatmeal with Hemp and Chia Seeds (page 61), Overnight Steel-Cut Oatmeal (page 60), Chia Pudding Power Bowl (page 62), or Buckwheat-Banana Pancakes (page 63). **Lunch:** Add ¼ teaspoon ground cinnamon to Creamy Mango Lassi (page 172) to enjoy alongside a lunch recipe from this book. **Dinner:** Add ½ teaspoon ground cinnamon to a serving of pear with sunflower seed butter to eat with a dinner recipe from this book.
ARTIFICIAL FOOD COLORING Note: It is challenging to find a food that contains only food dye. Using a rainbow fruit candy eliminates many of the eight major food allergens but does not eliminate everything. If you experience symptoms with any of these candy suggestions, reference your journal to see if you experienced symptoms with any other foods that may be ingredients in these candies. • SweeTarts • Skittles • Dots	**Breakfast:** Begin with 5 pieces of candy in the morning. **Lunch:** Increase to half a serving (according to candy package) at lunch. **Dinner:** Increase to 1 serving (according to candy package) at dinner.

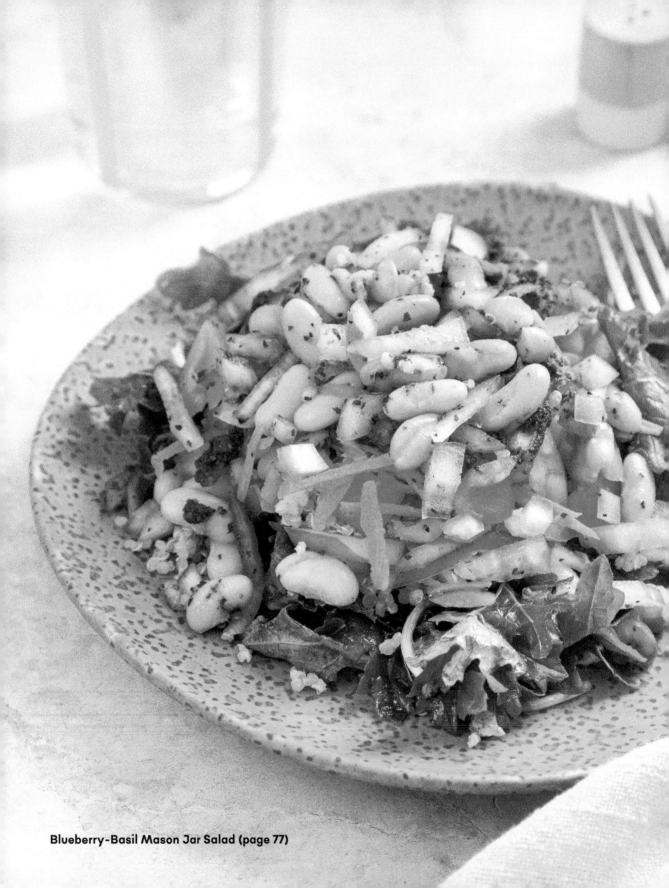

Blueberry-Basil Mason Jar Salad (page 77)

PART 3

The Recipes

ONE OF THE most challenging parts about completing an Elimination Diet is figuring out what you *can* eat when faced with an overwhelming list of everything that's off limits. The recipes in this book will take all the guesswork out of the equation and provide you with a variety of meals that are flavorful and enjoyable.

Note: I tested all recipes that call for sunflower seed butter with a natural, no-sugar-added sunflower seed butter that needs to be stirred due to a natural separation of the oil and seed butter.

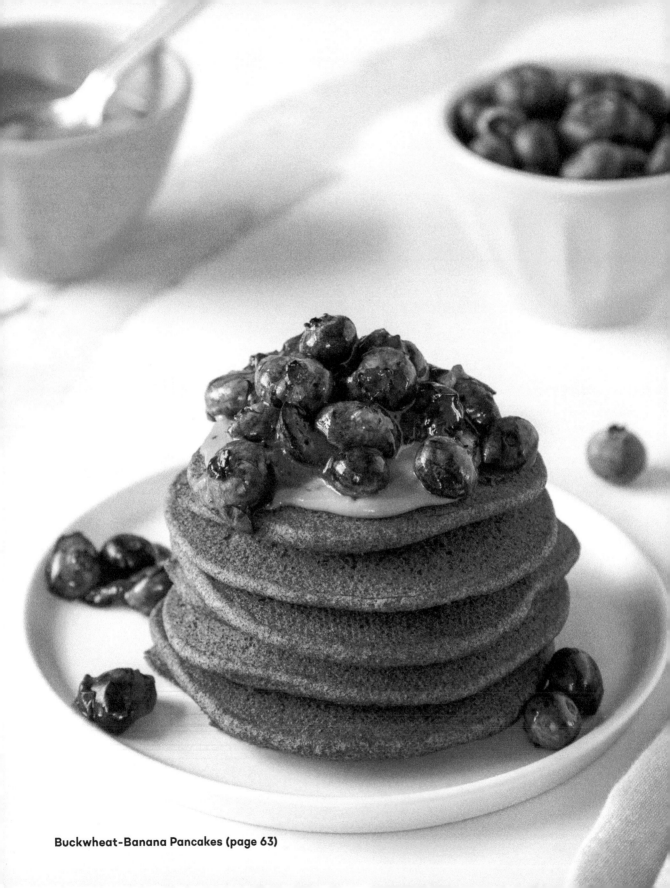

Buckwheat-Banana Pancakes (page 63)

CHAPTER 6

Breakfast

Overnight Steel-Cut Oatmeal

PREP TIME: 5 MINUTES, PLUS 6 HOURS TO THICKEN | COOK TIME: 5 MINUTES | YIELD: 4 SERVINGS

Steel-cut oats have a nutty flavor and chewy texture that is a little different from traditional oats. This recipe is great for busy seasons of life because you can "set it and forget it" and make breakfast for 4 (or 4 days) while you are sleeping.

1 cup steel-cut oats (certified gluten-free)

2 cups water

2 cups unsweetened rice, hemp, oat, or flax milk (check the ingredient list for any potential foods not allowed during the elimination phase)

Optional toppings: sunflower seed butter, shelled unsalted sunflower seeds (if you can only find salted, make sure there are no other ingredients that may cause a reaction, and adjust the salt as needed in the recipe), diced pear or any other fruit on the approved list, and/or maple syrup or agave syrup

1. Combine the oats, water, and milk in a large pot or Dutch oven. Bring to a boil over high heat and continue to boil for about 2 minutes, adjusting the heat as necessary to make sure it doesn't boil over.

2. Remove the pot from the heat source and cover. Let sit overnight, or for at least 6 hours, allowing the oats to cook and thicken up. Stir the thickened oats, reheat, and serve with your choice of toppings.

STORAGE: Store in an airtight container in the refrigerator for up to 4 days.

TIME-SAVER TIP: Schedule time to cook these oats while you are sleeping, so in the morning all you have to do is reheat, add your favorite toppings, and dig in.

PER SERVING (WITHOUT TOPPINGS): Calories: 162; Total fat: 3.5g; Total carbs: 32g; Fiber: 7g; Sugar: 0g; Protein: 6g; Sodium: 67mg

Banana Oatmeal with Hemp and Chia Seeds

PREP TIME: 5 MINUTES, PLUS 1 HOUR TO THICKEN | YIELD: 1 SERVING

Chia seeds are an amazing source of fiber and anti-inflammatory omega-3 fatty acids. They're also the secret ingredient in this oatmeal, because when liquid is added, they gel and expand, creating a creamy texture. This breakfast is subtly sweet and satisfying and will absolutely tide you over until lunch.

½ cup rolled or quick oats (certified gluten-free)

½ banana, mashed

1 cup unsweetened rice, hemp, oat, or flax milk (check the ingredient list for any potential foods not allowed during the elimination phase)

1 tablespoon flax meal

1 tablespoon chia seeds

1 tablespoon hemp seeds

1 teaspoon brown rice syrup, maple syrup, or agave syrup (optional)

Pinch kosher salt

Optional toppings: sliced banana and 1 tablespoon sunflower seed butter, or a handful of blueberries and 1 tablespoon sunflower seed butter

1. In a small food storage container or mason jar, combine the oats, banana, milk, flax, chia, hemp, brown rice syrup (if using), and salt. Stir to combine, cover, and refrigerate for at least 1 hour, or as long as overnight. When ready, the oats should be thick and soft.

2. Add the desired toppings and enjoy.

STORAGE: Store in an airtight container in the refrigerator for up to 4 days.

TIME-SAVER TIP: You can double or triple this batch to have breakfast ready ahead of time for later in the week.

PER SERVING (WITHOUT TOPPINGS): Calories: 423; Total fat: 16g; Total carbs: 66g; Fiber: 20g; Sugar: 13g; Protein: 14g; Sodium: 303mg

Chia Pudding Power Bowl

This light, refreshing bowl is filled with creamy and crunchy textures, sweet fruit, and a ton of staying power thanks to the fiber and nutritious fats in the chia seeds. Putting the chia and milk in the refrigerator the night before means the only thing you need to do in the morning is add toppings.

¼ cup chia seeds

1 cup unsweetened rice, hemp, oat, or flax milk (check the ingredient list for any potential foods not allowed during the elimination phase)

2 teaspoons maple syrup or agave syrup

Optional toppings: ¼ cup puffed rice cereal or puffed quinoa, 2 tablespoons blueberries, 1 peeled and diced kiwi, 2 tablespoons sunflower seed butter, and/or 1 teaspoon maple syrup or agave syrup

1. Combine the chia seeds, milk, and sweetener in a medium bowl and stir to combine. Cover and refrigerate for 1 hour. Stir the mixture, then cover and refrigerate for at least 6 hours, or overnight. This will allow the chia to gel and create a pudding consistency.

2. Divide the pudding between two bowls. Top each serving as desired.

STORAGE: Store in an airtight container in the refrigerator for up to 5 days.

PER SERVING (WITHOUT TOPPINGS): Calories: 160; Total fat: 7g; Total carbs: 19g; Fiber: 14g; Sugar: 4g; Protein: 6g; Sodium: 68mg

Buckwheat-Banana Pancakes

PREP TIME: 10 MINUTES | COOK TIME: 30 MINUTES | YIELD: 8 PANCAKES

Despite its name, buckwheat is not related to wheat at all and is naturally gluten-free. It is high in minerals as well as many antioxidants. Buckwheat's subtly sweet and nutty flavor makes it the perfect base for these simple and filling pancakes.

1 cup buckwheat flour

1 tablespoon flax meal

1 teaspoon baking soda

1/4 teaspoon kosher salt

1 cup unsweetened rice, hemp, oat, or flax milk (check the ingredient list for any potential foods not allowed during the elimination phase)

3 tablespoons canola oil, plus extra for the pan

2 tablespoons cane sugar

1 banana, sliced

1/2 cup blueberries

Sunflower seed butter, for topping

1. In a small bowl, whisk together the buckwheat flour, flax meal, baking soda, and salt. In a medium bowl, combine the milk, oil, and sugar. Add the dry ingredients to the wet ingredients, mixing just enough to combine them. Gently fold the sliced banana into the batter.

2. Heat a nonstick skillet over medium-high heat. Lightly coat the heated skillet with canola oil.

3. Pour about 1/4 cup of batter into the pan. Cook the first side for 1 to 2 minutes, until the top begins to bubble and the edges brown and dry out. Flip and cook the second side for another 1 to 2 minutes, until it can be easily lifted from the pan. The color will be darker than traditional pancakes because of the buckwheat flour. Repeat with the remaining batter.

4. Mash the blueberries in a small bowl with the back of a spoon or fork. Top each pancake with some sunflower seed butter and mashed blueberries.

STORAGE: Store extra pancakes in an airtight container in the refrigerator for up to 3 days, or freeze for up to 3 months. Reheat in the toaster or on the stove.

PER PANCAKE (WITHOUT TOPPINGS): Calories: 126; Total fat: 6g; Total carbs: 16g; Fiber: 4g; Sugar: 5g; Protein: 2g; Sodium: 247mg

Blueberry Breakfast Smoothie

PREP TIME: 5 MINUTES | YIELD: 2 SERVINGS

Hemp seeds are a wonderful source of plant-based protein. Paired with the fiber from the blueberries, hemp, and chia, this protein makes for a sweet and creamy smoothie that will power you through your morning. You'll want to keep some peeled ripe bananas in the freezer for this quick breakfast treat!

1½ cups unsweetened rice, hemp, oat, or flax milk (check the ingredient list for any potential foods not allowed during the elimination phase)

1 frozen banana

1½ cups frozen blueberries

2 tablespoons hemp seeds

1 tablespoon chia seeds

1 tablespoon sunflower seed butter

1 to 2 teaspoons maple syrup or agave syrup (optional)

Combine the unsweetened rice, hemp, oat, or flax milk; frozen banana; frozen blueberries; hemp seeds; chia seeds; sunflower seed butter; and maple syrup or agave syrup in a heavy-duty blender. Blend until smooth and creamy. Serve immediately.

TIME-SAVER TIP: Enjoying this smoothie alone? You can easily cut this recipe in half for a single serving.

PER SERVING: Calories: 290; Total fat: 12g; Total carbs: 42g; Fiber: 13g; Sugar: 19g; Protein: 8g; Sodium: 134mg

Tropical Green Smoothie

PREP TIME: 5 MINUTES | YIELD: 2 SERVINGS

The combination of kiwi, mango, and banana will make you feel like you're sipping this smoothie in warm, sunny weather no matter where you are. I added a hint of turmeric along with black pepper to enhance absorption of this anti-inflammatory spice, but don't worry—all you will taste is a sweet, creamy, delicious smoothie.

1½ cups unsweetened rice, hemp, oat, or flax milk (check the ingredient list for any potential ingredients not allowed during the elimination phase)

1 frozen banana

1 cup frozen mango chunks

1 kiwi, peeled

2 tablespoons hemp seeds

1 tablespoon flax meal

¼ teaspoon ground turmeric

Pinch ground black pepper

1 teaspoon maple syrup or agave syrup (optional)

Handful baby kale

Combine the unsweetened rice, hemp, oat, or flax milk; frozen banana; mango chunks; kiwi; hemp seeds; flax meal; turmeric; black pepper; maple syrup or agave syrup; and kale in a heavy-duty blender. Blend until smooth and creamy. Serve immediately.

PER SERVING: Calories: 255; Total fat: 8g; Total carbs: 47g; Fiber: 12g; Sugar: 25g; Protein: 7g; Sodium: 149mg

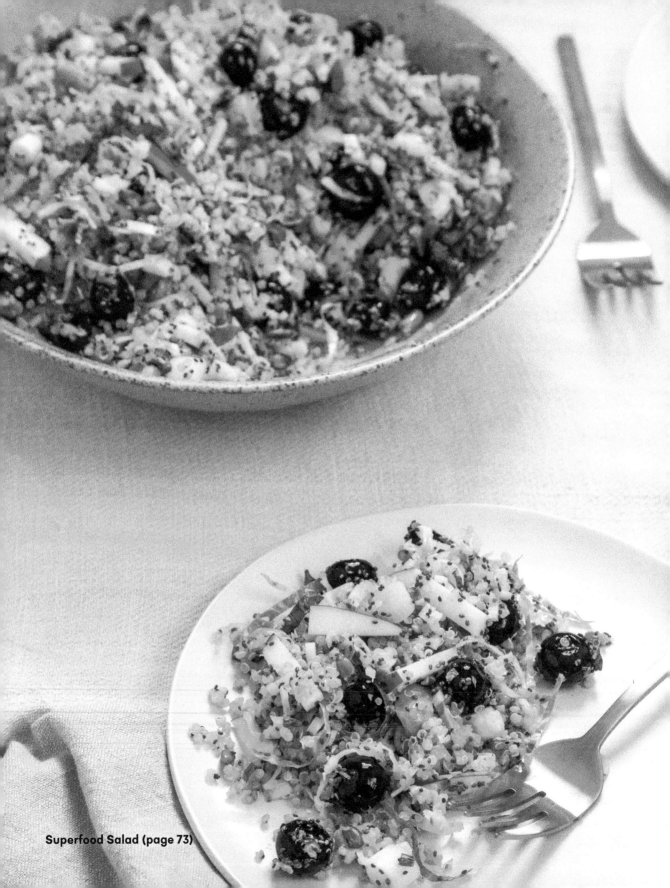

Superfood Salad (page 73)

CHAPTER 7

Salads and Bowls

Golden Roasted Cauliflower and Brown Rice Salad

PREP TIME: 20 MINUTES | COOK TIME: 20 MINUTES | YIELD: 2 MAIN-COURSE SERVINGS OR 4 SIDE-DISH SERVINGS

The gold color in this tasty dish comes from the bright yellow spice turmeric. Turmeric is high in curcumin, giving it anti-inflammatory and antioxidant properties, which are made more available to our bodies when paired with black pepper and healthy fats.

FOR THE CAULIFLOWER

1 head cauliflower, chopped

1 garlic clove, minced or grated

Canola oil cooking spray

1 teaspoon ground turmeric

1 teaspoon ground cumin

1 teaspoon paprika

1/4 teaspoon kosher salt

1/8 teaspoon ground black pepper

FOR THE DRESSING

3 tablespoons canola oil

1 tablespoon water

1 teaspoon sunflower seed butter

1 teaspoon maple syrup or
   agave syrup

1/8 teaspoon kosher salt

1/8 teaspoon ground turmeric

1/8 teaspoon ground cumin

1/8 teaspoon ground black pepper

FOR THE SALAD

3/4 cup cooked brown rice

1/2 (15-ounce) can white beans, rinsed
   and drained

1/4 cup shelled unsalted sunflower
   seeds (if you can only find salted,
   make sure there are no other
   ingredients that may cause a
   reaction, and adjust the salt as
   needed in the recipe)

1/4 cup chopped scallions

1. Preheat the oven to 425°F. Line a rimmed baking sheet with parchment paper or a silicone baking mat.

2. Scatter the cauliflower and garlic on the prepared baking sheet. Spritz with cooking spray. In a small bowl, combine the turmeric, cumin, paprika, salt, and pepper. Sprinkle over the cauliflower and toss with your hands to evenly coat. Spread out in a single

layer. Roast the cauliflower for about 20 minutes, until crisp and slightly brown. Let cool for about 10 minutes.

3. Combine the dressing ingredients in a jar with a tight-fitting lid. Shake to mix. (Alternatively, you can also whisk the ingredients together in a bowl.)

4. To assemble the salad, combine the roasted cauliflower, rice, beans, sunflower seeds, and scallions in a large bowl. Pour over the dressing, then toss until everything is well coated and combined. Serve and enjoy warm, at room temperature, or cold.

STORAGE: Store in an airtight container in the refrigerator for up to 5 days.

TIME-SAVER TIP: Make a batch of Simple Brown Rice (page 162) at the start of the week. Make the dressing and chop the vegetables a day ahead of time and store in the refrigerator.

PER SERVING (MAIN COURSE): Calories: 644; Total fat: 32g; Total carbs: 74g; Fiber: 22g; Sugar: 13g; Protein: 25g; Sodium: 641mg

Kitchen Sink Salad

PREP TIME: 20 MINUTES | COOK TIME: 20 MINUTES | YIELD: 2 SERVINGS

This salad includes everything except the kitchen sink! I love this recipe because it uses up any leftover vegetables and helps reduce food waste. You can stick with the vegetables I have listed below or sub in any vegetables you have on hand that are on the Foods You Can Eat list (pages 28–31).

FOR THE SALAD

1 cup chopped sweet potato or peeled butternut squash

5 Brussels sprouts, quartered

8 asparagus spears, trimmed and cut into 1-inch pieces

1 teaspoon canola oil

¼ teaspoon kosher salt

1 cup baby kale

1 cup thinly sliced cucumber rounds, cut in half

½ cup canned pinto beans

¼ cup shelled unsalted sunflower seeds (if you can only find salted, make sure there are no other ingredients that may cause a reaction, and adjust the salt as needed in the recipe)

FOR THE DRESSING

¼ cup unsweetened rice, hemp, oat, or flax milk (check the ingredient list for any potential foods not allowed during the elimination phase)

2 tablespoons sunflower seed butter

2 tablespoons water

2 teaspoons ground cumin

1 teaspoon ground turmeric

1 teaspoon paprika

¼ teaspoon ground black pepper

¼ teaspoon kosher salt

1 small garlic clove, minced

1. Preheat the oven to 425°F. Line a rimmed baking sheet with parchment paper or a silicone baking mat.

2. Scatter the sweet potato, Brussels sprouts, and asparagus on the prepared baking sheet, drizzle with the oil, and sprinkle with the salt. Roast for 20 to 25 minutes, until slightly crisp and brown.

3. While the vegetables roast, whisk together the dressing ingredients in a large bowl until smooth.

4. To assemble the salad, add the kale, cucumber, beans, sunflower seeds, and roasted vegetables to the bowl with the dressing. Toss until everything is well coated and mixed, then serve.

STORAGE: Store in an airtight container in the refrigerator for up to 5 days. Serve warm or cold.

PER SERVING: Calories: 391; Total fat: 19g; Total carbs: 43g; Fiber: 11g; Sugar: 8g; Protein: 14g; Sodium: 677mg

Sunflower White Bean Salad

PREP TIME: 10 MINUTES | YIELD: 3 SERVINGS

This is my take on a chicken or tuna salad. Since we are eliminating high-histamine and histamine-producing foods, consuming precooked meat is not currently an option. The sunflower seeds add a nice, crunchy texture, and the dill offers a fresh flavor that makes this white bean salad perfect for a midday meal.

1 (15-ounce) can white beans, rinsed and drained

¼ cup shelled unsalted sunflower seeds (if you can only find salted, make sure there are no other ingredients that may cause a reaction, and adjust the salt as needed in the recipe)

¼ cup chopped red onion

3 tablespoons sunflower seed butter

2 tablespoons finely chopped fresh dill, plus more for garnish

1 tablespoon maple syrup or agave syrup

1 teaspoon water

½ teaspoon paprika

¼ teaspoon kosher salt

Pinch ground black pepper

6 or 8 large cabbage leaves

½ cucumber, thinly sliced

1 bell pepper (any color), seeded and chopped

1. Lightly mash the beans in a medium bowl with the back of a fork or spoon. Add the sunflower seeds, onion, butter, dill, maple syrup, water, paprika, salt, and pepper. Mix to combine.

2. Place 2 cabbage leaves on each plate to use as "cups." Divide the cucumber and bell pepper among them, then top with the bean salad. Garnish with dill and serve.

STORAGE: Store in an airtight container in the refrigerator for up to 5 days.

PER SERVING: Calories: 322; Total fat: 14g; Total carbs: 38g; Fiber: 10g; Sugar: 6g; Protein: 14g; Sodium: 270mg

Superfood Salad

PREP TIME: 20 MINUTES | COOK TIME: 15 MINUTES | YIELD: 2 MAIN-COURSE SERVINGS OR 4 SIDE-DISH SERVINGS

This superfood salad is also super flavorful! I love pairing it with a protein to make it a meal. It's a simple salad to make, so I usually make it toward the start of the week to save time and enjoy for a few days.

FOR THE SALAD

½ cup quinoa

1 cup water

2 cups Brussels sprouts

1 cup blueberries

½ apple, cored and cut into matchsticks

¼ cup shelled unsalted sunflower seeds (if you can find only salted, make sure there are no other ingredients that may cause a reaction, and adjust the salt as needed in the recipe)

½ cup chopped scallions

¼ cup chia seeds

FOR THE DRESSING

¼ cup canola oil

2 tablespoons water

1 teaspoon minced or grated fresh ginger

½ teaspoon maple syrup or agave syrup

1 tablespoon chopped fresh chives

1 tablespoon chopped fresh basil (about 2 large leaves)

¼ teaspoon kosher salt

⅛ teaspoon ground turmeric

⅛ teaspoon ground black pepper

Pinch cayenne pepper

1. Combine the quinoa and water in a medium saucepan. Cover and bring to a boil over high heat. Reduce the heat to low and simmer for 10 to 15 minutes, until the water is absorbed and the quinoa is done. You will know it is ready when the germ starts to separate from the seed, with a little white curl coming off the main round part. Set aside.

2. Trim off the bottoms of the Brussels sprouts, then cut in half lengthwise. Place them cut-side down and thinly slice them into shreds.

3. Combine the quinoa, Brussels sprouts, blueberries, apple, sunflower seeds, scallions, and chia seeds in a large salad bowl.

> **CONTINUED ON NEXT PAGE**

Superfood Salad

> CONTINUED

4. Combine the dressing ingredients in a jar with a tight-fitting lid. Shake to mix. (Alternatively, you can whisk the ingredients together in a bowl.) Pour the dressing over the salad and toss until well coated and combined.

STORAGE: Store in an airtight container in the refrigerator for up to 5 days. Serve cold.

PER SERVING (MAIN COURSE): Calories: 734; Total fat: 44g; Total carbs: 72g; Fiber: 22g; Sugar: 17g; Protein: 19g; Sodium: 332mg

Herby Cauliflower Salad

PREP TIME: 20 MINUTES | COOK TIME: 30 MINUTES | YIELD: 4 SERVINGS

This raw cauliflower salad pairs sweet and savory in the best way possible. Filled with vibrant, fresh herbs, it makes for a great side dish to accompany any of the main dishes in this book or all on its own.

FOR THE SALAD

1 (15-ounce) can white beans, rinsed and drained

2 teaspoons canola oil

1 teaspoon paprika

1 teaspoon ground cumin

½ teaspoon kosher salt

¼ teaspoon ground black pepper

1 head cauliflower, cut into florets

1 apple, cored and thinly sliced

¼ cup finely chopped red onion

½ cup chopped fresh chives

½ cup chopped fresh basil

2 tablespoons chopped fresh oregano

FOR THE DRESSING

½ cup canola oil

½ cup water

2 tablespoons chopped fresh chives

1 teaspoon dried basil

1 teaspoon dried oregano

1 teaspoon kosher salt

¼ teaspoon ground black pepper

1. Preheat the oven to 400°F. Line a rimmed baking sheet with parchment paper or a silicone baking mat.

2. Put the beans on the prepared baking sheet and drizzle with the oil. In a small bowl, mix the paprika, cumin, salt, and pepper, then sprinkle evenly over the beans. Spread out in a single layer. Roast for 20 to 30 minutes, until slightly crisp and brown.

3. Working in batches, pulse the cauliflower in a food processor until it has the texture of rice. Transfer to a large bowl.

4. Combine all the dressing ingredients in a jar with a tight-fitting lid. Shake to mix. (Alternatively, you can whisk the ingredients together in a bowl.)

5. To assemble the salad, add the roasted beans, apple, onion, and fresh herbs to the cauliflower rice. Pour over the dressing and toss until everything is well coated and combined. Enjoy warm, at room temperature, or cold.

STORAGE: Store in an airtight container in the refrigerator for up to 5 days.

PER SERVING: Calories: 423; Total fat: 30g; Total carbs: 32g; Fiber: 11g; Sugar: 9g; Protein: 10g; Sodium: 936mg

Fresh Greens and Blueberry Salad with Easy Dill Dressing

PREP TIME: 10 MINUTES | YIELD: 2 SERVINGS

Meet your new go-to side salad! Sweet blueberries are the perfect contrast to the unique flavor of dill. It's a simple recipe, so you can easily make it in the evening while your main dish is cooking.

FOR THE SALAD

¼ cup shelled unsalted sunflower seeds (if you can find only salted, make sure there are no other ingredients that may cause a reaction, and adjust the salt as needed in the recipe)

3 cups baby kale

⅓ cup blueberries

½ cup diced cucumber

FOR THE DRESSING

3 tablespoons canola oil

2 tablespoons chopped fresh dill, plus extra for garnish

3 tablespoons water

¼ teaspoon kosher salt

Ground black pepper

1. In a dry nonstick skillet, toast the sunflower seeds over medium heat for about 5 minutes, stirring occasionally, until they become fragrant. Remove from the heat.
2. Combine all the dressing ingredients in a jar with a tight-fitting lid. Shake to mix. (Alternatively, you can also whisk the ingredients together in a bowl.)
3. Divide the kale between two bowls, then top each bowl with the toasted sunflower seeds, blueberries, and cucumber. Pour the dressing over each salad and toss to combine. Garnish with dill and serve.

STORAGE: Store the dressing and the salad separately in airtight containers in the refrigerator for up to 5 days.

PER SERVING: Calories: 305; Total fat: 29g; Total carbs: 8g; Fiber: 3g; Sugar: 4g; Protein: 4g; Sodium: 314mg

Blueberry-Basil Mason Jar Salad

PREP TIME: 20 MINUTES | YIELD: 4 SERVINGS

Blueberry and basil are a match made in heaven. We use whole blueberries in this dressing to get all the benefits of this sweet summer berry. You'll find that this is a delicious dressing for almost any kind of salad.

FOR THE DRESSING

1 cup blueberries

¾ cup packed fresh basil leaves

½ cup water

1 teaspoon maple syrup or agave syrup

1 teaspoon dried oregano

1 garlic clove, peeled

½ teaspoon kosher salt

¼ teaspoon ground black pepper

FOR THE SALAD

½ small red onion, diced

1 (15-ounce) can pinto beans or white beans, rinsed and drained

1 bell pepper (any color), seeded and chopped

1 large carrot, peeled and grated

1 cup Perfectly Cooked Quinoa (page 163), cooled

4 cups baby kale

1. Combine all the dressing ingredients in a blender or food processor and blend until smooth.

2. To assemble the salads, set 4 wide-mouth quart-size mason jars on your counter. Pour equal amounts of the dressing into the bottom of each container. On top of the dressing, layer the onion, beans, bell pepper, carrot, quinoa, and kale, in that order. (Putting the dressing on the bottom will keep the vegetables from getting soggy.)

3. Close the jars and refrigerate until you are ready to serve.

4. To serve, pour the contents of each jar into a large bowl. The dressing will now be on top of the salad. Stir to combine and enjoy!

STORAGE: Store in an airtight container in the refrigerator for up to 4 days.

PER SERVING: Calories: 196; Total fat: 1g; Total carbs: 38g; Fiber: 8g; Sugar: 8g; Protein: 9g; Sodium: 469mg

Mediterranean Mason Jar Pesto Salad

PREP TIME: 20 MINUTES TOTAL | YIELD: 4 SERVINGS

This delicious recipe lets you spend less than 30 minutes in the kitchen to enjoy a fresh and flavorful midday meal.

FOR THE DRESSING

½ cup packed fresh basil leaves

1 garlic clove, peeled

1 tablespoon shelled unsalted sunflower seeds (if you can find only salted, make sure there are no other ingredients that may cause a reaction, and adjust the salt as needed in the recipe)

1 tablespoon hemp seeds

½ teaspoon kosher salt

¼ cup canola oil

¼ cup water

FOR THE SALAD

½ small red onion, diced

1 English cucumber, diced

1 (15-ounce) can white beans, rinsed and drained

1 bell pepper (any color), seeded and chopped

1 head romaine lettuce, trimmed and chopped

½ cup shelled unsalted sunflower seeds (if you can find only salted, make sure there are no other ingredients that may cause a reaction, and adjust the salt as needed in the recipe)

1. Pulse the basil and garlic in a food processor until chopped. Add the sunflower and hemp seeds and salt and pulse again until finely chopped and mixed. With the machine running, slowly pour in the oil through the feed tube until thickened. Stop the food processor and scrape down the sides as necessary. Add 1 tablespoon of water at a time to thin as needed.

2. To assemble the salads, set 4 wide-mouth quart-size mason jars on your counter. Pour equal amounts of the dressing into the bottom of each jar. On top of the dressing, layer the diced onion, cucumber, beans, bell pepper, romaine, and sunflower seeds, in that order. (Putting the dressing on the bottom will help prevent the vegetables from getting soggy.)

3. Close the jars and refrigerate until you are ready to serve.

4. To serve, pour the contents of each jar into a large bowl. The dressing will now be on top. Stir to combine and enjoy!

PER SERVING: Calories: 374; Total fat: 24g; Total carbs: 31g; Fiber: 10g; Sugar: 6g; Protein: 13g; Sodium: 305mg

Roasted Vegetable and Brown Rice Bowl with Green Sauce

PREP TIME: 15 MINUTES | COOK TIME: 35 MINUTES | YIELD: 4 SERVINGS

Roasting vegetables makes them crisp and brown on the outside and tender on the inside, and it really enhances the flavor. If you aren't a fan of a particular vegetable, give it a try roasted. I suggest one of my favorite combinations of vegetables for this recipe, but you can use any vegetables you have on hand; just refer to the Foods You Can Eat list (pages 28–31).

FOR THE ROASTED VEGETABLES

6 cups chopped vegetables (I like this combo: 4 small carrots, 1 medium potato, 1 small zucchini, and 8 asparagus spears)

1 tablespoon canola oil

1/2 teaspoon kosher salt

FOR THE BROWN RICE

1 cup brown rice

2 cups water

FOR THE SAUCE

1/2 cup loosely packed fresh chives

2 garlic cloves, peeled

3 tablespoons hemp seeds

1/2 teaspoon kosher salt

6 tablespoons canola oil

1/2 cup water, or more as needed

1. Preheat the oven to 400°F. Line a rimmed baking sheet with parchment paper or a silicone baking mat.

2. In a large bowl, toss the chopped vegetables with the oil and salt. Arrange in a single layer on the prepared baking sheet and roast for about 30 minutes, until the vegetables are brown and crisp.

3. While the vegetables are roasting, combine the rice and water in a medium saucepan, cover, and bring to a boil over high heat. Reduce the heat to low and simmer for about 35 minutes, until all the water is absorbed. Set aside.

4. To make the sauce, pulse the chives and garlic together in a food processor until finely chopped. Add the hemp seeds and salt and pulse until finely chopped and mixed. With the machine running, slowly pour the oil through the feed tube and process until thickened. Stop the food processor and scrape down the sides as necessary. Add 1 tablespoon of water at a time to thin as needed.

5. Divide the rice and vegetables between four bowls, top with the sauce, and serve.

STORAGE: Store in an airtight container in the refrigerator for up to 5 days.

PER SERVING: Calories: 481; Total fat: 29g; Total carbs: 50g; Fiber: 6g; Sugar: 5g; Protein: 9g; Sodium: 621mg

Sweet Potato Buddha Bowl

PREP TIME: 15 MINUTES | COOK TIME: 35 MINUTES | YIELD: 4 SERVINGS

A Buddha bowl is a vegetarian meal served in a bowl filled with lots of different foods. Here we have roasted broccoli and sweet potato, brown rice, and a mouthwatering sunflower seed butter dressing, creating a meal that will make you shine from the inside out.

FOR THE ROASTED VEGETABLES

1 head broccoli, cut into florets
  (about 2 cups)
2 cups cubed sweet potatoes
1 garlic clove, minced
1 tablespoon canola oil
1/4 teaspoon kosher salt
1/8 teaspoon ground black pepper

FOR THE RICE

1 cup brown rice
2 cups water
1 teaspoon ground cumin
1/4 teaspoon kosher salt
1/4 teaspoon canola oil

FOR THE DRESSING

1/4 cup sunflower seed butter
1/4 cup water
1 teaspoon canola oil
1 teaspoon maple syrup or
  agave syrup
1 garlic clove, minced

1 tablespoon minced or grated peeled
  fresh ginger
1 teaspoon onion powder (make sure
  it's all natural, with no additives)
1/4 teaspoon kosher salt

FOR THE GARNISH

1 cup chopped scallions

1. Preheat the oven to 425°F. Line a rimmed baking sheet with parchment paper or a silicone baking mat.

2. On the baking sheet, toss the broccoli and sweet potatoes with the garlic, oil, salt, and pepper. Spread out in a single layer and roast for about 30 minutes, until brown and crisp.

3. While the vegetables are roasting, combine the rice and water in a medium saucepan, cover, and bring to a boil. Reduce the heat to low and simmer for about 35 minutes, until all the water is absorbed, then stir in the cumin, salt, and oil.

4. In a small bowl, whisk together all the dressing ingredients until smooth.

5. Divide the seasoned rice into four bowls. Top with the roasted broccoli and sweet potatoes, drizzle with the sunflower seed butter dressing, sprinkle with the scallions, and serve.

STORAGE: Store in an airtight container in the refrigerator for up to 5 days. You can serve warm or cold.

TIME-SAVER TIP: Make the sauce and chop the vegetables one day ahead of time and refrigerate.

PER SERVING: Calories: 403; Total fat: 15g; Total carbs: 61g; Fiber: 7g; Sugar: 7g; Protein: 10g; Sodium: 521mg

Sweet Potato Falafel Bowl

PREP TIME: 20 MINUTES | COOK TIME: 15 MINUTES | YIELD: 4 SERVINGS

Traditional falafel gets a makeover! Instead of a bean base, this take on the Mediterranean classic has sweet potatoes as its foundation. Sweet potatoes are rich in antioxidants like beta-carotene, which is converted to vitamin A in the body. Vitamin A is great for boosting your immune system, skin health, and eye health.

FOR THE SWEET POTATO FALAFEL

1 small sweet potato, chopped (about 1 cup)

1 cup cooked brown rice

1/2 cup shelled unsalted sunflower seeds (if you can find only salted, make sure there are no other ingredients that may cause a reaction, and adjust the salt as needed in the recipe)

1 tablespoon roughly chopped fresh chives

1 flax egg (see page 85)

1 teaspoon kosher salt

1/2 cup rolled oats (certified gluten-free), ground in a food processor to a flour-like texture

6 to 7 tablespoons canola oil

FOR THE DRESSING

1/2 cup loosely packed fresh chives

2 garlic cloves, peeled

3 tablespoons hemp seeds

1 teaspoon ground cumin

1/2 teaspoon kosher salt

1/2 jalapeño pepper, seeded

6 tablespoons canola oil

1/2 cup water

FOR THE BOWLS

4 cups torn red and green cabbage

1 cup cooked brown rice or quinoa

1 cup chopped cucumber

1 cup chopped bell pepper

1. To make the falafel, pulse the sweet potato in a food processor until the pieces are very small. Add the brown rice, sunflower seeds, and chives and pulse until combined and all the sweet potato pieces look similar in size. Add the flax egg and pulse until fully mixed in. Transfer the mixture to a bowl and stir in the salt and ground oats. Form the mixture into 16 even balls and slightly flatten them.

2. Heat the oil in a large nonstick skillet over medium heat until shimmering. Working in batches, panfry the falafel for about 2 minutes per side, until golden brown and cooked through. (Alternatively, you can roast the falafel on a rimmed baking sheet at 400°F for about 20 minutes, until crisp on the outside and slightly golden brown.)

3. To make the dressing, pulse the chives and garlic in a food processor until finely chopped. Add the hemp seeds, cumin, and salt and pulse until finely chopped and mixed. Add the jalapeño and pulse until finely chopped and mixed. With the machine running, slowly pour the oil through the feed tube and process until thickened. Stop the food processor and scrape down the sides as necessary. Add 1 tablespoon of water at a time to thin as needed.

4. Divide the cabbage, rice, cucumber, and bell pepper into four bowls. Add the dressing and mix to combine. Top each bowl of dressed vegetables with 4 falafel and serve.

STORAGE: Store in an airtight container in the refrigerator for up to 5 days. Reheat the falafel prior to serving.

PER SERVING: Calories: 738; Total fat: 56g; Total carbs: 51g; Fiber: 10g; Sugar: 7g; Protein: 12g; Sodium: 897mg

HOW TO MAKE A FLAX EGG

Here is a great, egg-free alternative when you need a binder in a recipe. For each large egg, combine 1 tablespoon ground flax meal with 2½ tablespoons water. Allow to sit on the counter for about 5 minutes to thicken and gel.

Bell Pepper and Basil Wild Rice Bowl

PREP TIME: 10 MINUTES | COOK TIME: 1 HOUR | YIELD: 2 SERVINGS

This meal-size bowl is full of bright, fresh flavor thanks to a pesto created just for this book. Crunchy kale is massaged to give it a more tender texture, and sweet bell peppers add just the right amount of crunch.

FOR THE WILD RICE

⅓ cup wild rice, rinsed and drained
1⅓ cups water
Pinch kosher salt

FOR THE BOWL

2 cups torn stemmed kale leaves
¼ teaspoon kosher salt
¼ teaspoon canola oil
½ bell pepper (any color), seeded and diced
¼ cup Basil Pesto (page 121)

1. Combine the rice, water, and salt in a medium saucepan and bring to a boil over high heat. Reduce the heat to low, cover, and simmer for 45 to 55 minutes, until the rice is tender but still a little chewy. Drain off any remaining liquid.

2. Put the kale in a medium bowl and rub the salt and oil into the leaves to soften them.

3. Divide the kale, bell pepper, and wild rice between two bowls. Top with the pesto dressing and enjoy.

STORAGE: Store the components separately in airtight containers in the refrigerator for up to 5 days. You can serve warm or cold.

TIME-SAVER TIP: Use baby kale and you can skip step 2. Make the wild rice in a large batch and freeze in individual portions, or make a smaller batch one day ahead of time and refrigerate.

PER SERVING: Calories: 402; Total fat: 26g; Total carbs: 33g; Fiber: 5g; Sugar: 1g; Protein: 9g; Sodium: 684mg

Roasted Cauliflower Quinoa Bowl

Cauliflower is packed with vitamins and minerals, and quinoa is filled with plant protein. So this cauliflower-quinoa combo makes for a yummy, nutrient-packed meal that's really simple to make.

FOR THE ROASTED CAULIFLOWER

1 head cauliflower, cut into florets
1 garlic clove, minced
1 tablespoon canola oil
½ teaspoon ground turmeric
¼ teaspoon kosher salt
¼ teaspoon ground black pepper

FOR THE QUINOA

1 cup quinoa
2 cups water
¼ cup chopped scallions
¼ teaspoon kosher salt
¼ teaspoon canola oil

FOR THE DRESSING

¼ cup canola oil
2 tablespoons water
1 garlic clove, minced
½ teaspoon paprika
½ teaspoon kosher salt
¼ teaspoon ground black pepper

1. Preheat the oven to 400°F. Line a rimmed baking sheet with parchment paper or a silicone baking mat.

2. Toss the cauliflower with the garlic, oil, turmeric, salt, and pepper and spread out in a single layer on the prepared baking sheet. Roast for about 30 minutes, until the cauliflower is brown and crisp.

3. While the cauliflower is roasting, combine the quinoa and water in a medium saucepan, cover, and bring to a boil. Reduce the heat to low and simmer for 10 to 15 minutes, until all the water is absorbed and the quinoa is done. You will know it is ready when the germ starts to separate from the seed, with a little white curl coming off the main round part. Stir in the scallions, salt, and oil. Whisk all the dressing ingredients together in a small bowl.

> CONTINUED ON NEXT PAGE

Roasted Cauliflower Quinoa Bowl

> CONTINUED

4. Divide the seasoned quinoa into four bowls. Top with the roasted cauliflower and drizzle with the dressing. Adjust the seasoning by adding more salt, pepper, and/or garlic to taste.

STORAGE: Store in an airtight container in the refrigerator for up to 5 days. You can serve warm or cold.

PER SERVING: Calories: 383; Total fat: 21g; Total carbs: 43g; Fiber: 8g; Sugar: 7g; Protein: 10g; Sodium: 647mg

Meal Prep Quinoa Taco Bowl

PREP TIME: 10 MINUTES | COOK TIME: 15 MINUTES | YIELD: 4 SERVINGS

"Meal prep" is a trendy term for cooking ahead of time to make eating nutritious food later in the week a whole lot simpler. This salad fits the bill. You can easily toss this together quickly on a weekend and have lunch ready to go all week.

1 cup quinoa

2 cups water

1 (15-ounce) can pinto beans, rinsed
   and drained

1 cup chopped bell pepper (any color)

1 cup shredded red or green cabbage

½ cup chopped scallions

1 jalapeño pepper, seeded
   and chopped

2 teaspoons ground cumin

½ teaspoon kosher salt

1 tablespoon canola oil

1. Combine the quinoa and water in a medium saucepan and bring to a boil over high heat. Reduce the heat to low, cover, and simmer for 10 to 15 minutes, until the water is absorbed and the quinoa is done. You will know it is ready when the germ starts to separate from the seed, with a little white curl coming off the main round part. Remove from the heat, uncover, and let cool for 10 minutes.

2. In a large bowl, combine the cooked quinoa, beans, bell pepper, cabbage, scallions, jalapeño, cumin, salt, and oil. Toss to combine, adjusting the seasoning as needed.

3. Divide into four bowls and enjoy.

STORAGE: Store in an airtight container in the refrigerator for up to 5 days.

TIME-SAVER TIP: Chop the vegetables one day ahead of time and refrigerate.

PER SERVING: Calories: 304; Total fat: 6g; Total carbs: 50g; Fiber: 8g; Sugar: 6g; Protein: 12g; Sodium: 298mg

Spring Roll Bowl

PREP TIME: 15 MINUTES | COOK TIME: 15 MINUTES | YIELD: 4 SERVINGS

I put a fun twist on classic spring rolls by swapping rice noodles for rice paper and tossing the noodles and veggies with a yummy herb sauce. This dish is packed with vibrant color and fresh, herby flavor. Add the chicken only if you are serving this dish immediately. If you plan on making it in advance, omit the chicken. Leftover chicken has a greater chance of being high in histamines, which is something we want to avoid during the elimination phase.

FOR THE CHICKEN (OPTIONAL)

1 pound boneless, skinless chicken breasts, cut into bite-size pieces
1 teaspoon canola oil
1 small garlic clove, minced or grated
¼ teaspoon kosher salt
¼ teaspoon ground black pepper

FOR THE RICE NOODLES

7 ounces rice noodles

FOR THE SAUCE

¼ cup chopped fresh chives
¼ cup chopped fresh basil
2 garlic cloves, peeled
3 tablespoons hemp seeds
1 tablespoon shelled unsalted sunflower seeds (if you can find only salted, make sure there are no other ingredients that may cause a reaction, and adjust the salt as needed in the recipe)

½ teaspoon kosher salt
6 tablespoons canola oil
½ cup water

FOR THE BOWLS

1 cup chopped fresh basil
½ cup cucumber strips
½ cup chopped red cabbage
1 carrot, cut into matchsticks
½ bell pepper (any color), seeded and cut into thin strips
¼ cup shelled unsalted sunflower seeds (if you can find only salted, make sure there are no other ingredients that may cause a reaction, and adjust the salt as needed in the recipe)
Red pepper flakes

1. If using the chicken, preheat the oven to 425°F. Line a rimmed baking sheet with parchment paper or a silicone baking mat.
2. Toss the chicken with the oil, garlic, salt, and black pepper, spread out on

the prepared baking sheet in a single layer, and bake for about 15 minutes, until cooked through.

3. Meanwhile, prepare the rice noodles according to the package instructions. Typically, this requires soaking them in boiling water to soften. Drain.

4. Pulse the chives, basil, and garlic in a food processor until finely chopped. Add the hemp seeds, sunflower seeds, and salt and pulse until finely chopped and mixed. With the machine running, slowly pour the oil through the feed tube and process until thickened. Stop the food processor and scrape down the sides as necessary. Add 1 tablespoon of water at a time to thin as needed.

5. Combine the rice noodles with about half of the dressing in a large bowl. Add the basil, cucumber, cabbage, carrot, bell pepper, sunflower seeds, chicken (if using), and red pepper flakes to taste. Toss to combine. Divide into four bowls and top each bowl with the remaining dressing.

STORAGE: Store (without the chicken) in an airtight container in the refrigerator for up to 5 days.

PER SERVING (WITH CHICKEN): Calories: 615; Total fat: 34g; Total carbs: 48g; Fiber: 3g; Sugar: 2g; Protein: 32g; Sodium: 646mg

PER SERVING (WITHOUT CHICKEN): Calories: 307; Total fat: 9g; Total carbs: 47g; Fiber: 3g; Sugar: 2g; Protein: 9g; Sodium: 466mg

Soba Noodle Bowl with Chicken and Sunflower Sauce

PREP TIME: 10 MINUTES | COOK TIME: 15 MINUTES | YIELD: 4 SERVINGS

Soba noodles are made with buckwheat flour, which despite its name has no relation to the wheat that we are avoiding during the elimination phase. (You'll want to read the label on your package of noodles to make sure "buckwheat" is the only ingredient.) This traditional Japanese noodle cooks up quickly and has a slightly nutty flavor and a very soft texture. If you find that you love the sauce, double the recipe and add extra to your bowls. Any leftover sauce tastes great with fresh vegetable dippers!

FOR THE CHICKEN

1 pound boneless, skinless chicken breast, cut into bite-size pieces
1 small garlic clove, minced or grated
1 teaspoon canola oil
¼ teaspoon kosher salt
¼ teaspoon ground black pepper

FOR THE SAUCE

¼ cup sunflower seed butter
6 tablespoons warm water
1 tablespoon canola oil
1 garlic clove, minced or grated
2 teaspoons chopped fresh or freeze-dried chives
¼ teaspoon kosher salt
¼ teaspoon red pepper flakes

FOR THE BOWLS

8 ounces soba noodles (check the package to make sure the only ingredient is buckwheat)
2 cups diced cucumber
2 cups shredded green or red cabbage

1. Preheat the oven to 425°F. Line a rimmed baking sheet with parchment paper or a silicone baking mat.
2. Toss the chicken with the garlic, oil, salt, and black pepper, spread out on the prepared baking sheet, and bake for about 15 minutes, until cooked through.
3. While the chicken is cooking, prepare the sauce. Whisk together the sunflower seed butter, water, oil, garlic, chives, salt, and red pepper flakes until smooth. Set aside.

4. Cook the noodles according to the package directions. Drain and rinse with cold water to stop the cooking process. Return the noodles to the pot that you cooked them in and toss with half the sauce.

5. Divide the noodles with sauce into four bowls. Top each bowl with an equal amount of cucumber, cabbage, and cooked chicken. Drizzle with the remaining sauce (you may need to add a couple tablespoons of water to thin it). Serve immediately; the dish will be a combination of warm and cold, crunchy and soft.

STORAGE: Store (without the chicken) in an airtight container in the refrigerator for up to 5 days.

MAKE IT MEATLESS: If you omit the chicken and can tolerate soy products, cubed tofu or tempeh would taste delicious in this dish!

PER SERVING: Calories: 459; Total fat: 16g; Total carbs: 50g; Fiber: 2g; Sugar: 4g; Protein: 36g; Sodium: 990mg

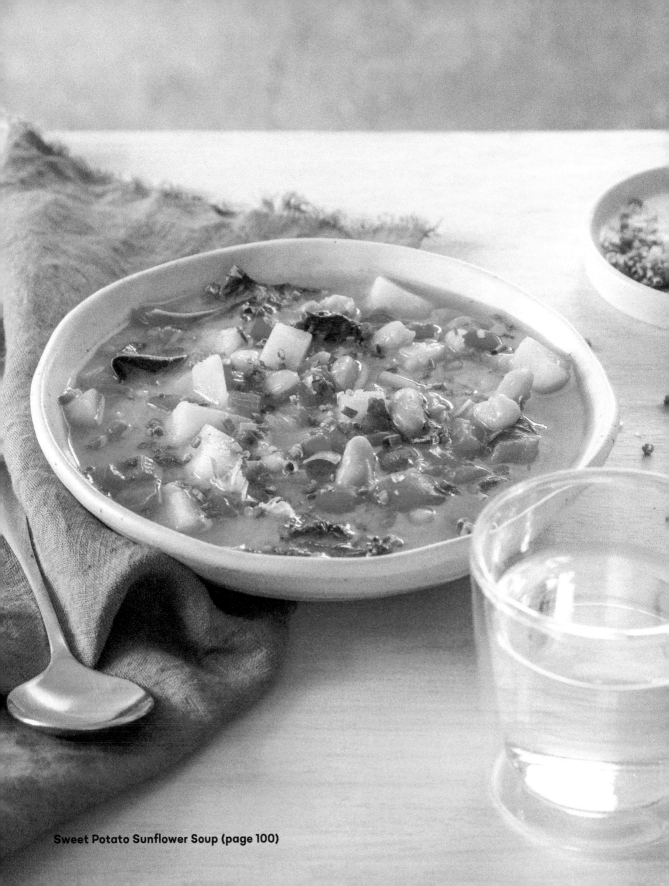

Sweet Potato Sunflower Soup (page 100)

CHAPTER 8

Soups, Stews, and Chili

Allergy-Free Broth

This simple broth recipe is rich in flavor and adds a ton of depth to many of the dishes in this book. Traditional store-bought broths may contain ingredients we are removing during the elimination phase, so this is a great recipe to make on the weekend to use in recipes throughout the week.

2 to 4 cups veggie scraps from the week (kale stems, carrot tops, onion peels, zucchini ends, etc.)

1 carrot, roughly chopped

5 fresh chives

½ onion, roughly chopped

2 teaspoons kosher salt

1 teaspoon ground black pepper

8 cups water

1. Combine all the ingredients in a large pot or Dutch oven. Cover and bring to boil over high heat. Reduce the heat to low and simmer for about 3 hours.

2. Taste and adjust the seasoning of the broth. Remove from the heat and let cool to room temperature. Strain (discard the solids) before using or storing.

STORAGE: Store in airtight containers in the refrigerator for up to 4 days or in the freezer for up to 6 months. When freezing the broth, I like to freeze it in ice cube trays with 1 to 2 tablespoons in each slot so I can easily measure how much broth I am adding.

PER SERVING: Calories: 6; Total fat: 0g; Total carbs: 1g; Fiber: 0g; Sugar: 1g; Protein: 0g; Sodium: 587mg

Chicken Soup with Quinoa and Greens

PREP TIME: 15 MINUTES | COOK TIME: 30 MINUTES | YIELD: 4 SERVINGS

The combination of carbohydrates (vegetables and quinoa), protein (chicken and quinoa), and fat (canola oil) makes this meal extremely filling—and the addition of fresh dill at the end adds a zippy flavor.

FOR THE CHICKEN

- 1 pound boneless, skinless chicken breast
- 1 garlic clove, lightly smashed
- 1 tablespoon roughly chopped fresh oregano
- ¼ onion, roughly chopped
- ½ teaspoon kosher salt
- 6 cups water

FOR THE SOUP

- 2 teaspoons canola oil
- 2 medium carrots, diced
- ½ onion, diced
- 2 garlic cloves, minced
- ¾ cup quinoa
- 1 handful baby kale or regular kale
- 1 teaspoon kosher salt
- ¼ teaspoon ground black pepper
- ¼ cup chopped fresh dill

1. Combine all the ingredients for the chicken in a large saucepan, cover, and bring to a simmer over medium heat. Reduce the heat to low and cook for 10 to 14 minutes, until the chicken is cooked through. Strain and reserve the poaching liquid. Shred the chicken with two forks.

2. To make the soup, heat the oil in a medium saucepan over medium heat. Add the carrots, onion, and garlic and cook for about 5 minutes, stirring frequently until soft.

3. Add the reserved poaching liquid and quinoa and bring to a boil. Cover, reduce the heat to low, and simmer for 10 to 15 minutes, until the quinoa is done. You will know it is ready when the germ starts to separate from the seed, with a little white curl coming off the main round part.

> **CONTINUED ON NEXT PAGE**

Chicken Soup with Quinoa and Greens

> CONTINUED

4. Add the shredded chicken, kale, salt, pepper, and dill and serve.

> **STORAGE:** If you are sensitive to histamines or completing the elimination phase, bring the soup to room temperature, then store it in an airtight container in the freezer for up to 4 months. When you are ready to enjoy leftovers, thaw and reheat to an internal temperature of 165°F. If you are not sensitive to histamines, store in an airtight container in the refrigerator for up to 4 days.

PER SERVING: Calories: 314; Total fat: 7g; Total carbs: 32g; Fiber: 4g; Sugar: 5g; Protein: 32g; Sodium: 1,188mg

Creamy Golden Soup

PREP TIME: 10 MINUTES | COOK TIME: 25 MINUTES | YIELD: 4 SERVINGS

This soup has a velvety texture and simple flavor that make it perfect to enjoy on a rainy day. The star ingredients include vitamin- and mineral-rich cauliflower and anti-inflammatory turmeric.

1½ tablespoons canola oil

½ onion, chopped

2 small garlic cloves, chopped

1 head cauliflower, cut into florets

¾ cup shelled unsalted sunflower seeds (if you can find only salted, make sure there are no other ingredients that may cause a reaction, and adjust the salt as needed in the recipe)

2 teaspoons ground turmeric

6 cups water

1¼ teaspoons kosher salt

½ teaspoon ground black pepper

1. Heat the oil in a large pot or Dutch oven. Add the onion, garlic, cauliflower, sunflower seeds, and turmeric and cook for about 10 minutes, stirring occasionally.

2. Add the water, salt, and pepper and bring to a boil. Cover, reduce the heat to low, and simmer for about 10 minutes, until the cauliflower is soft.

3. Use an immersion blender to purée the soup in the pot or let the soup cool a bit, then carefully transfer it in batches to a blender or food processor and blend until creamy. Reheat and serve.

STORAGE: Store in an airtight container in the refrigerator for up to 4 days or in the freezer for up to 6 months.

PER SERVING: Calories: 250; Total fat: 18g; Total carbs: 19g; Fiber: 8g; Sugar: 5g; Protein: 9g; Sodium: 792mg

Sweet Potato Sunflower Soup

PREP TIME: 15 MINUTES | COOK TIME: 15 MINUTES | YIELD: 4 SERVINGS

Here's a twist on one of my favorite soups. Creamy and a little spicy, this soup will quickly become a favorite of yours, too.

1 teaspoon canola oil

3 tablespoons chopped fresh chives

1 garlic clove, minced

1 red bell pepper, seeded and chopped

1 jalapeño pepper, seeded and minced

1 medium sweet potato, diced

½ teaspoon kosher salt

¼ teaspoon ground black pepper

4½ cups Allergy-Free Broth
     (page 96), divided

⅓ cup sunflower seed butter

2 teaspoons ground cumin

1 teaspoon paprika

¼ teaspoon cayenne pepper

1 (15-ounce) can white beans, rinsed
     and drained

2 large handfuls baby kale or
     regular kale

1. Heat the oil in a large pot or Dutch oven over medium heat. Add the chives, garlic, bell pepper, jalapeño, sweet potato, salt, black pepper, and ½ cup of broth. Increase the heat to medium-high and boil gently for about 5 minutes.

2. In a medium bowl, combine the sunflower seed butter and 1 cup of broth. Stir until creamy and smooth. Add this mixture and the remaining 3 cups of broth to the pot, then stir in the cumin, paprika, and cayenne. Cover and bring to a boil. Reduce the heat to low and simmer for 10 minutes. The sweet potatoes should fall apart when pierced with a fork.

3. Add the beans and kale. Stir to combine and serve.

STORAGE: Store in an airtight container in the refrigerator for up to 4 days.

PER SERVING: Calories: 300; Total fat: 12g; Total carbs: 36g; Fiber: 8g; Sugar: 6g; Protein: 12g; Sodium: 1051mg

Butternut Squash and White Bean Soup

PREP TIME: 10 MINUTES | COOK TIME: 30 MINUTES | YIELD: 2 SERVINGS

Butternut squash and white beans make this soup extremely velvety, and the cumin gives it a bit of smoky flavor. Butternut squash is like pumpkin's cousin and a great source of vitamin A, and white beans are high in potassium, fiber, B vitamins and plant protein, making this a dish packed with nutrients and flavor.

2 to 3 cups chopped peeled butternut squash

3 teaspoons canola oil, divided

2 teaspoons ground cumin

¼ teaspoon red pepper flakes (optional)

2 cups unsweetened rice, hemp, oat, or flax milk (check the ingredient list for any potential foods not allowed during the elimination phase)

1 cup water

1 cup Allergy-Free Broth (page 96)

1 (15-ounce) can white beans, rinsed and drained

½ teaspoon kosher salt (optional)

¼ teaspoon ground black pepper

1. Preheat the oven to 425°F. Line a rimmed baking sheet with parchment paper or a silicone baking mat.

2. Toss the squash with 1 teaspoon of oil and spread in a single layer on the prepared baking sheet. Roast for about 25 minutes, until slightly browned on the outside and tender on the inside.

3. Heat the remaining 2 teaspoons of oil in a medium saucepan over medium heat. Add the cumin and red pepper flakes (if using) and stir until fragrant. Add the milk, water, and broth and bring to a boil.

4. Add the roasted squash, beans, salt, and black pepper and let heat through for several minutes. Use an immersion blender to purée the soup in the pot or let it cool a bit, then transfer it in batches to a blender or food processor and purée until smooth. Reheat and serve.

STORAGE: If there are leftovers, let the soup cool for at least 10 minutes, then transfer to an airtight container and store in the refrigerator for up to 4 days or in the freezer for up to 4 months.

PER SERVING: Calories: 377; Total fat: 11g; Total carbs: 62g; Fiber: 20g; Sugar: 6g; Protein: 13g; Sodium: 438mg

Sweet Potato Zoodle Soup with Creamy Turmeric Sauce

PREP TIME: 10 MINUTES | COOK TIME: 30 MINUTES | YIELD: 2 SERVINGS

Zucchini spirals act like noodles in this dish, making it a fun and tasty way to add extra vegetables. The sauce is extremely creamy but free of dairy and any other potential allergens.

½ teaspoon canola oil

1 garlic clove, minced

1 teaspoon minced or grated peeled fresh ginger

½ small white onion, diced

½ bell pepper (any color), seeded and diced

1 medium sweet potato, diced

1 teaspoon ground turmeric

1 cup unsweetened rice, hemp, oat, or flax milk (check the ingredient list for any potential foods not allowed during the elimination phase)

1 tablespoon sunflower seed butter

¼ teaspoon kosher salt

¼ teaspoon ground black pepper

1 medium zucchini, spiralized into noodles

Cayenne pepper (optional)

1. In a large soup pot or Dutch oven, heat the oil over medium-high heat. Add the garlic and ginger and cook for 1 to 2 minutes, stirring, until fragrant. Add the onion, bell pepper, and sweet potato and cook for about 10 minutes, stirring occasionally, until softened. Add the turmeric and stir to coat the vegetables.

2. Add the milk, sunflower seed butter, salt, and black pepper. Stir until everything is combined. Bring the mixture to a boil, then reduce the heat to low and simmer for about 10 minutes, stirring occasionally, until the sweet potatoes are fork-tender.

3. Stir the zucchini noodles into the soup and simmer for about 3 minutes to heat through. Stir in cayenne to taste (if using). Ladle into two bowls and enjoy.

STORAGE: If there are leftovers, let the soup to cool for at least 10 minutes, then transfer to an airtight container and store in the refrigerator for up to 4 days or in the freezer for up to 4 months. Thaw and reheat prior to serving.

TIME-SAVER TIP: You can find already spiralized zucchini in the produce section of many supermarkets.

PER SERVING: Calories: 188; Total fat: 7g; Total carbs: 30g; Fiber: 7g; Sugar: 7g; Protein: 5g; Sodium: 406mg

Beef Stew

PREP TIME: 15 MINUTES | COOK TIME: 3 HOURS | YIELD: 4 SERVINGS

A simple makeover on a classic dish results in the perfect meal for the elimination phase in this book.

1 tablespoon canola oil

1 pound boneless beef chuck, tip, or round roast, cut into bite-size pieces

1 small white onion, diced

3 cups Allergy-Free Broth (page 96)

1 teaspoon kosher salt, or more to taste

¼ teaspoon ground black pepper, or more to taste

2 medium carrots, peeled and cut into 1-inch pieces

1 large russet potato, peeled and cut into 1-inch pieces

1 green bell pepper, seeded and roughly chopped

1. In a large soup pot or Dutch oven, heat the oil over medium heat. When it shimmers, add the beef and brown it on all sides for about 8 minutes total.

2. Add the onion and cook for about another 8 minutes, stirring occasionally, until translucent. Add the broth, salt, and pepper and bring to a boil. Cover, reduce the heat to low, and simmer for about 2 hours, until the beef is nearly tender.

3. Stir in the carrots, potato, and bell pepper, raise the heat to medium, and bring to a boil. Cover, reduce the heat to low, and simmer for about 30 minutes, until the potatoes are fork-tender.

4. Taste the broth and season with more salt and pepper if necessary.

STORAGE: If you are sensitive to histamines or completing the elimination phase, allow leftovers to cool for at least 10 minutes, then store them in an airtight container in the freezer for up to 4 months. When you are ready to enjoy leftovers, thaw and reheat to an internal temperature of 165°F. If you are not sensitive to histamines, store leftovers in an airtight container in the refrigerator for up to 4 days.

PER SERVING: Calories: 393; Total fat: 24g; Total carbs: 22g; Fiber: 4g; Sugar: 4g; Protein: 24g; Sodium: 998mg

White Bean Turkey Chili

This tomato-free chili is filled with smoky cumin flavor.

2 teaspoons canola oil

1/2 medium white onion, diced

2 garlic cloves, minced

1 jalapeño pepper, seeded and minced

1/2 teaspoon kosher salt, divided

1/4 teaspoon ground black pepper

1 pound ground turkey (93% lean)

2 teaspoons ground cumin

1/2 teaspoon dried oregano

2 cups Allergy-Free Broth (page 96)

1 1/2 (15-ounce) cans Great Northern beans, rinsed and drained, divided

1. In a large soup pot or Dutch oven, heat the oil over medium heat. Add the onion, garlic, jalapeño, 1/4 teaspoon of salt, and the pepper. Cook for about 8 minutes, stirring occasionally, until softened, reducing the heat to medium-low if the vegetables start browning.

2. Add the turkey, cumin, and oregano and cook for about 5 minutes, breaking up the turkey with your spoon or spatula, until the meat is no longer pink. Add the broth and bring to a simmer.

3. Mash the half can of beans in a small bowl with a fork or spoon until mostly smooth. Add it and the whole beans to the chili, along with the remaining 1/4 teaspoon of salt. Stir to combine. Bring the chili to a boil, then cover, reduce the heat to low, and simmer for 10 minutes. Serve and enjoy.

STORAGE: If you are sensitive to histamines or completing the elimination phase, allow leftovers to cool for at least 10 minutes, then store them in an airtight container in the freezer for up to 4 months. When you are ready to enjoy leftovers, thaw and reheat to an internal temperature of 165°F. If you are not sensitive to histamines, store in an airtight container in the refrigerator for up to 4 days.

PER SERVING: Calories: 315; Total fat: 10g; Total carbs: 25g; Fiber: 6g; Sugar: 2g; Protein: 30g; Sodium: 670mg

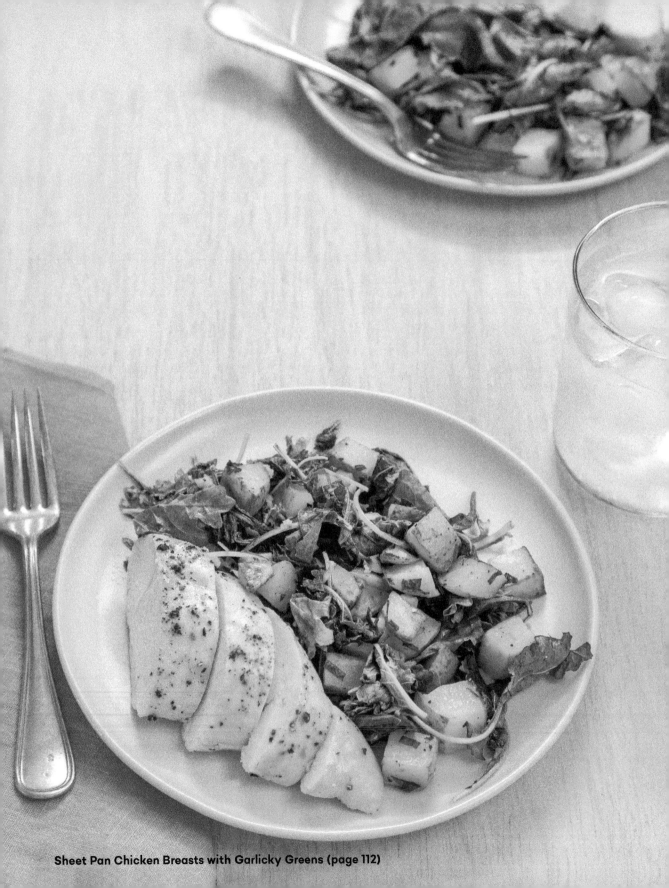

Sheet Pan Chicken Breasts with Garlicky Greens (page 112)

CHAPTER 9

Chicken

Slow Cooker Chicken Quinoa Primavera

PREP TIME: 15 MINUTES | COOK TIME: 4½ HOURS | YIELD: 4 SERVINGS

Pasta Primavera is traditionally made with lightly sautéed spring vegetables. Here, I pair the spring vegetables with pesto and toss them in the slower cooker with quinoa and chicken to make a super creamy one-pot dish.

½ pound boneless, skinless chicken breast

¾ cup quinoa

2 garlic cloves, minced

1 teaspoon dried oregano

1 teaspoon dried basil

½ teaspoon kosher salt

¼ teaspoon ground black pepper

2 to 3½ cups Allergy-Free Broth (page 96), divided

¼ cup Basil Pesto (page 121)

1 cup frozen peas

10 asparagus spears, trimmed and chopped

½ cup chopped fresh chives

1. Combine the chicken, quinoa, garlic, oregano, basil, salt, pepper, and 2 cups of broth in the slow cooker. Cover and cook on low for 4 hours.

2. If the consistency is very thick and sticky, slowly stir in the remaining 1½ cups of broth, ½ cup at a time, until you have a nice, creamy texture. Transfer the chicken to a cutting board and shred it with two forks, then return it to the cooker.

3. Stir in the pesto, peas, and asparagus, cover, and cook for 30 more minutes on low.

4. Sprinkle with the chives and serve.

STORAGE: If you are sensitive to histamines or completing the elimination phase, allow leftovers to cool for at least 10 minutes, then store them in an airtight container in the freezer for up to 4 months. When you are ready to enjoy leftovers, thaw and reheat to an internal temperature of 165°F. If you are not sensitive to histamines, store leftovers in an airtight container in the refrigerator for up to 4 days.

MAKE IT MEATLESS: Substitute one (15-ounce) can of white beans, rinsed and drained, for the meat, adding them at the end with the pesto, peas, and asparagus.

PER SERVING: Calories: 370; Total fat: 18g; Total carbs: 33g; Fiber: 6g; Sugar: 6g; Protein: 21g; Sodium: 1083mg

Slow Cooker
Maple-Garlic Chicken

PREP TIME: 5 MINUTES | COOK TIME: 2 TO 4 HOURS ON HIGH OR 6 TO 8 HOURS ON LOW |
YIELD: 4 SERVINGS

I adore using the slow cooker throughout the year. It's great in the winter for warm, comforting food, and it's ideal in the summer when It's too hot to turn on the stove or oven. This dish has an Asian flavor thanks to the spicy ginger and sweet maple, making it perfect for any season. I like to serve it with Garlic-Ginger Bok Choy (page 159) and Simple Brown Rice (page 162).

3 garlic cloves, minced

1 (1-inch) piece fresh ginger, peeled and minced or grated

½ cup water

⅓ cup maple syrup

¾ teaspoon kosher salt

¼ teaspoon red pepper flakes (optional)

1 pound boneless, skinless chicken breast

1½ teaspoons potato starch

1. In a small bowl, whisk together the garlic, ginger, water, maple syrup, salt, and red pepper flakes (if using) until the maple syrup is mostly dissolved.

2. Put the chicken in the slow cooker, then pour the sauce over the chicken. Cover and cook on high for 2 to 4 hours or low for 6 to 8 hours.

3. Transfer the chicken to a cutting board and shred it using two forks. Stir the potato starch into the sauce. Return the chicken to the cooker, stir to coat with the sauce, cover, and cook on low for about 10 more minutes, so the sauce can thicken, then serve.

STORAGE: If you are sensitive to histamines or completing the elimination phase, allow leftovers to cool for at least 10 minutes, then store them in an airtight container in the freezer for up to 4 months. When you are ready to enjoy leftovers, thaw and reheat to an internal temperature of 165°F. If you are not sensitive to histamines, store leftovers in an airtight container in the refrigerator for up to 4 days.

PER SERVING: Calories: 187; Total fat: 3g; Total carbs: 19g; Fiber: 0g; Sugar: 16g; Protein: 23g; Sodium: 619mg

One-Pot Italian Chicken with Rice and Vegetables

PREP TIME: 15 MINUTES | COOK TIME: 50 MINUTES | YIELD: 4 SERVINGS

I love how easy cleanup is after prepping a one-pot meal. This easy dish includes vegetables, whole grains, protein, and some of my favorite Italian spices (basil and oregano).

1 tablespoon canola oil, divided

1 pound boneless, skinless chicken breast, cut into bite-size pieces

1/2 white onion, diced

2 medium carrots, peeled and diced

3 garlic cloves, minced

2 teaspoons dried oregano

1 teaspoon dried basil

2 1/2 cups Allergy-Free Broth (page 96)

1 cup brown rice

1/2 medium head cauliflower, cut into florets

1/2 cup frozen green peas

1. In a large pot, heat the oil over medium-high heat. Add the chicken and brown for about 5 minutes per side. Transfer the chicken to a plate.

2. Add the onion and carrots to the pot and cook for about 5 minutes, stirring occasionally, until slightly softened. Add the garlic, oregano, and basil and cook for about a minute, stirring, until fragrant. Add the broth, rice, cauliflower, and chicken and stir to combine. Bring to a boil, cover, reduce the heat to low, and simmer for about 30 minutes, until the rice is tender.

3. Remove from the heat and stir in the frozen peas. Cover and let stand for 5 minutes to let the peas heat up, then serve.

STORAGE: If you are sensitive to histamines or completing the elimination phase, allow leftovers to cool for at least 10 minutes, then store them in an airtight container in the freezer for up to 4 months. When you are ready to enjoy leftovers, thaw and reheat to an internal temperature of 165°F. If you are not sensitive to histamines, store leftovers in an airtight container in the refrigerator for up to 4 days.

PER SERVING: Calories: 367; Total fat: 8g; Total carbs: 48g; Fiber: 7g; Sugar: 5g; Protein: 31g; Sodium: 838mg

Roasted Turmeric Chicken with Broccoli

PREP TIME: 10 MINUTES | COOK TIME: 25 MINUTES | YIELD: 2 SERVINGS

Bright-yellow turmeric is high in curcumin, which is a strong antioxidant that also has anti-inflammatory properties. Not only is this vibrant, bright green-and-yellow meal stunning to look at, it's also made in one dish, so cleanup's a breeze.

½ **pound boneless, skinless chicken breast, cut into 4 pieces**

2 **teaspoons ground turmeric**

2 **teaspoons canola oil**

1 **medium head broccoli, cut into florets**

2 **small garlic cloves, minced**

2 **tablespoons maple syrup**

½ **teaspoon kosher salt**

¼ **teaspoon ground black pepper**

1. Preheat the oven to 400°F.

2. Sprinkle the chicken with the turmeric. Heat the oil in a large oven-safe skillet over high heat. Add the chicken and pan-sear for about 2 minutes on each side. Remove the pan from the heat, add the broccoli and garlic, and drizzle with the maple syrup. The pan will seem very full, but the broccoli will cook down in size.

3. Transfer the pan to the oven and bake for about 10 minutes, until the chicken is cooked through.

4. Sprinkle with the salt and pepper and serve.

STORAGE: If you are sensitive to histamines or completing the elimination phase, allow leftovers to cool for at least 10 minutes, then store them in an airtight container in the freezer for up to 4 months. When you are ready to enjoy leftovers, thaw and reheat to an internal temperature of 165°F. If you are not sensitive to histamines, store leftovers in an airtight container in the refrigerator for up to 4 days.

TIME-SAVER TIP: Chop the broccoli ahead of time and let it sit before cooking, which allows sulforaphane compounds to develop. Sulforaphane is a plant compound in cruciferous vegetables that may benefit heart health and digestion.

PER SERVING: Calories: 298; Total fat: 8g; Total carbs: 31g; Fiber: 10g; Sugar: 17g; Protein: 32g; Sodium: 846mg

Sheet Pan Chicken Breasts with Garlicky Greens

PREP TIME: 15 MINUTES | COOK TIME: 40 MINUTES | YIELD: 4 SERVINGS

In my house, sheet pan meals are essential for busy weeknights. This dish comes together quickly and needs only about 30 minutes in the oven—just enough time to complete any last-minute to-dos before getting dinner on the table.

4 Yukon Gold potatoes, cut into 1-inch cubes

2 tablespoons chopped fresh oregano

2 tablespoons chopped fresh chives

2 teaspoons canola oil

½ teaspoon kosher salt, divided

½ teaspoon ground black pepper, divided

½ pound boneless, skinless chicken breast

5 cups stemmed kale

4 garlic cloves, minced or grated

1. Preheat the oven to 375°F. Line a rimmed baking sheet with parchment paper or a silicone baking mat.

2. In a medium bowl, toss the potatoes, oregano, chives, oil, ¼ teaspoon of salt, and ¼ teaspoon of pepper together until well mixed. Spread out in a single layer on the prepared baking sheet, leaving enough space in the center for the chicken.

3. Season the chicken with the remaining ¼ teaspoon of salt and ¼ teaspoon of pepper and place in the center of the pan, not on top of the potatoes. Bake for about 30 minutes, until the chicken is cooked through.

4. Remove the pan from the oven and transfer the chicken to a plate. Add the kale and garlic to the sheet pan and toss with the potatoes. Roast for about 10 more minutes, until the kale starts to crisp.

5. Divide the potatoes, greens, and chicken between two plates and serve.

STORAGE: If you are sensitive to histamines or completing the elimination phase, allow leftovers to cool for at least 10 minutes, then store them in an airtight container in the freezer for up to 4 months. When you are ready to enjoy leftovers, thaw and reheat to an internal temperature of 165°F. If you are not sensitive to histamines, store leftovers in an airtight container in the refrigerator for up to 4 days.

TIME-SAVER TIP: Use baby kale instead of regular kale; it will yield a more tender though less crisp result.

PER SERVING: Calories: 236; Total fat: 4g; Total carbs: 36g; Fiber: 5g; Sugar: 3g; Protein: 18g; Sodium: 419mg

Chicken with Chimichurri

PREP TIME: 15 MINUTES | COOK TIME: 25 MINUTES | YIELD: 2 SERVINGS

Chimichurri is a fresh green herb sauce typically used when seasoning meat. This version uses oregano and basil, giving it a bright flavor. To make the chimichurri, I find it easiest to put all the herbs in a large pile and chop them together, constantly adjusting them on the cutting board so everything is chopped. Pair this with Simple Brown Rice (page 162), Simple Roasted Vegetables (page 156), or Kiwi Green Salsa (page 161).

FOR THE CHICKEN

½ pound boneless, skinless
   chicken breast
Canola oil cooking spray
¼ teaspoon ground cumin
¼ teaspoon kosher salt
Pinch ground black pepper

FOR THE CHIMICHURRI

½ cup finely chopped fresh oregano
½ cup finely chopped fresh basil
2 tablespoons finely chopped
   red onion
1 garlic clove, minced
¼ teaspoon kosher salt
Pinch red pepper flakes
2 tablespoons canola oil
3 tablespoons water

1. Preheat the oven to 425°F. Line a rimmed baking sheet with parchment paper or aluminum foil and spritz with cooking spray.

2. Place the chicken on the prepared baking sheet and spritz with the spray. In a small bowl, combine the cumin, salt, and black pepper, then sprinkle the spice mixture over the top of the chicken. Roast for 20 to 25 minutes, until cooked through.

3. Combine all the chimichurri ingredients in a bowl. Stir to combine, then adjust the flavors as necessary.

> **CONTINUED ON NEXT PAGE**

Chicken with Chimichurri

> CONTINUED

4. Divide the chicken into two portions. Top with the chimichurri and serve.

STORAGE: If you are sensitive to histamines or completing the elimination phase, allow leftovers to cool for at least 10 minutes, then store them in an airtight container in the freezer for up to 4 months. When you are ready to enjoy leftovers, thaw and reheat to an internal temperature of 165°F. If you are not sensitive to histamines, store leftover chicken in an airtight container in the refrigerator for up to 4 days and leftover chimichurri in a separate container for up to 1 day.

TIMER-SAVER TIP: You can make the chimichurri a day ahead, which will allow the flavors to meld.

PER SERVING: Calories: 245; Total fat: 17g; Total carbs: 2g; Fiber: 1g; Sugar: 0g; Protein: 24g; Sodium: 763mg

Warm Herby Chicken and Rice Bowl

PREP TIME: 20 MINUTES | COOK TIME: 1 HOUR | YIELD: 2 SERVINGS

This dish is extremely comforting and perfect for a cold, gray day. Blending the sunflower seeds, canola oil, and water makes a creamy, oh-so-satisfying dressing.

FOR THE RICE:

- ½ cup wild rice or wild rice blend (make sure the only ingredients are different varieties of rice without added flavoring), rinsed and drained
- 1½ cups water

FOR THE CHICKEN:

- ½ pound boneless, skinless chicken breast, cut into bite-size pieces
- 1 teaspoon canola oil
- ¼ teaspoon kosher salt
- ¼ teaspoon ground black pepper
- 1 garlic clove, minced or grated
- 2 cups chopped red bell pepper (about 1 bell pepper)

FOR THE DRESSING

- ¾ cup canola oil
- ½ cup shelled unsalted sunflower seeds (if you can find only salted, make sure there are no other ingredients that may cause a reaction, and adjust the salt as needed in the recipe)
- ½ cup water
- ½ cup packed fresh basil leaves
- ½ cup packed fresh oregano leaves
- 1 garlic clove, peeled
- 1 teaspoon kosher salt

1. Combine the rice and water in a medium saucepan and bring to a boil over high heat. Reduce the heat to low, cover, and simmer for 45 to 55 minutes, until the rice is tender but still a little chewy. Drain off any remaining liquid.

2. Meanwhile, preheat the oven to 425°F. Line a rimmed baking sheet with parchment paper or a silicone baking mat.

3. In a medium bowl, toss the chicken with the oil, salt, pepper, and garlic. Arrange on the prepared baking sheet and bake for about 15 minutes, until cooked through.

4. Pulse all the dressing ingredients in a food processor until smooth and creamy.

> **CONTINUED ON NEXT PAGE**

Warm Herby Chicken and Rice Bowl

> CONTINUED

5. Combine the rice, chicken, and bell pepper in a large bowl. Toss with 5 tablespoons of the dressing and season to taste as necessary. Divide between two plates and enjoy with any remaining dressing offered on the side.

STORAGE: If you are sensitive to histamines or completing the elimination phase, allow leftovers to cool for at least 10 minutes, then store them in an airtight container in the freezer for up to 4 months. When you are ready to enjoy leftovers, thaw and reheat to an internal temperature of 165°F. If you are not sensitive to histamines, store leftovers, with the dressing in a separate container, in the refrigerator for up to 4 days.

TIME-SAVER TIP: Cook the rice ahead of time and refrigerate in an airtight container for up to 4 days.

MAKE IT MEATLESS: If you are not allergic or sensitive to soy products, after completing the elimination phase, you can replace the chicken with tofu or tempeh. If you are not sensitive to histamines, you can use lentils in place of the chicken.

PER SERVING: Calories: 1257; Total fat: 103g; Total carbs: 54g; Fiber: 8g; Sugar: 5g; Protein: 37g; Sodium: 1638mg

Asparagus-Stuffed Chicken Breasts

PREP TIME: 20 MINUTES | COOK TIME: 30 MINUTES | YIELD: 2 SERVINGS

This dish is gorgeous enough for a special occasion but simple enough to enjoy on a busy weeknight. Flattening the chicken makes it simple to roll around the nutritious (and, dare I say, stunning) asparagus.

Canola oil cooking spray

2 boneless, skinless chicken breasts (½ pound total)

1 tablespoon dried oregano

¼ teaspoon kosher salt

⅛ teaspoon ground black pepper

8 asparagus spears, trimmed

1 tablespoon canola oil

2 garlic cloves, minced

1. Preheat the oven to 375°F. Line a rimmed baking sheet with parchment paper or aluminum foil and spritz with cooking spray.

2. Place one chicken breast in a zip-top plastic bag, then use a mallet, rolling pin, cutting board, can of food, or plastic bottle of water to pound the chicken to ¼-inch thickness. Repeat with the other chicken breast. Sprinkle the chicken breasts on both sides with the oregano, salt, and pepper.

3. Place 4 asparagus spears in the center of each chicken breast and roll the chicken around them. You may need to use toothpicks to help keep the chicken together. Place the rolled chicken breasts seam-side down on the prepared baking sheet.

4. In a small bowl, whisk together the oil and garlic and drizzle over the chicken. Bake for 25 to 30 minutes, until the chicken is cooked through. Remove the toothpicks before serving.

STORAGE: If you are sensitive to histamines or completing the elimination phrase, allow leftovers to cool for at least 10 minutes, then store them in an airtight container in the freezer for up to 4 months. When you are ready to enjoy leftovers, thaw and reheat to an internal temperature of 165°F. If you are not sensitive to histamines, store leftovers in an airtight container in the refrigerator for up to 4 days.

PER SERVING: Calories: 198; Total fat: 10g; Total carbs: 5g; Fiber: 2g; Sugar: 1g; Protein: 25g; Sodium: 473mg

Chicken Cauliflower Skillet

Cauliflower is one of the few vegetables that have nearly every vitamin and mineral in it, which makes it the perfect, nutritious base for this one-dish meal.

½ pound boneless, skinless chicken breast

½ teaspoon kosher salt

⅛ teaspoon ground black pepper

1 teaspoon canola oil

½ cup Allergy-Free Broth (page 96)

2 cups chopped cauliflower

2 garlic cloves, minced

1 tablespoon chopped fresh basil

1 tablespoon unsweetened rice, hemp, oat, or flax milk (check the ingredient list for any potential foods not allowed during the elimination phase)

1. Season the chicken on both sides with the salt and pepper. Heat the oil in a large skillet over medium-high heat. Add the chicken and cook for 3 to 5 minutes per side, until golden brown. Transfer the chicken to a plate.

2. Add the broth, cauliflower, garlic, and basil to the skillet and stir, scraping up any browned bits from the bottom of the pan. Cook for about 5 minutes, until the liquid is almost completely reduced and the cauliflower is tender-crisp.

3. Remove the skillet from the heat and stir in the milk. Return the chicken to the pan and simmer it all together for 5 minutes, then serve.

STORAGE: If you are sensitive to histamines or completing the elimination phase, allow leftovers to cool for at least 10 minutes, then store them in an airtight container in the freezer for up to 4 months. When you are ready to enjoy leftovers, thaw and reheat to an internal temperature of 165°F. If you are not sensitive to histamines, store leftovers in an airtight container in the refrigerator for up to 4 days.

TIME-SAVER TIP: Make a batch of broth at the start of the week to use in recipes throughout the week.

PER SERVING: Calories: 162; Total fat: 5g; Total carbs: 7g; Fiber: 3g; Sugar: 2g; Protein: 25g; Sodium: 939mg

Garlic Skillet Chicken

PREP TIME: 5 MINUTES | COOK TIME: 15 MINUTES | YIELD: 2 SERVING

Garlic lovers, this is for you! Some of my favorite sides to partner with this
Dilled Bean Salad with Carrots and Quinoa (page 152), Roasted Brussels S
with Wild Rice (page 157), and Mediterranean Roasted Asparagus (page 155).
I like to get all the ingredients for the side dish measured and chopped first, then
I prepare the side dish as the chicken cooks.

3 teaspoons canola oil, divided

1 garlic clove, minced

**1/2 teaspoon maple syrup or
   agave syrup**

1/4 teaspoon dried oregano

Pinch red pepper flakes (optional)

**2 boneless, skinless chicken breasts
   (about 1/2 pound)**

1/4 teaspoon kosher salt

1/8 teaspoon ground black pepper

1. In a small bowl, whisk together
   2 teaspoons of oil, the garlic, maple
   syrup, oregano, and red pepper flakes
   (if using).

2. Season the chicken on both sides with
   the salt and black pepper, then heat
   the remaining 1 teaspoon of oil in a
   large skillet over medium-high heat.
   Pan-sear the chicken for 3 to 4 minutes
   on the first side. Flip the chicken and
   drizzle it with the garlic-oregano oil.
   Reduce the heat to medium and cook
   the chicken for 8 to 10 more minutes,
   until cooked through, then serve.

STORAGE: If you are sensitive to histamines
or completing the elimination phase, allow
leftovers to cool for at least 10 minutes, then
store them in an airtight container in the
freezer for up to 4 months. When you are
ready to enjoy leftovers, thaw and reheat to
an internal temperature of 165°F. If you are
not sensitive to histamines, store leftovers
in an airtight container in the refrigerator for
up to 4 days.

PER SERVING: Calories: 176; Total fat: 9g;
Total carbs: 2g; Fiber: 0g; Sugar: 1g; Protein: 23g;
Sodium: 471mg

Mango Chicken

PREP TIME: 15 MINUTES | COOK TIME: 25 MINUTES | YIELD: 2 SERVINGS

Have you ever tried fruit salsa? Sweet and spicy salsa pairs perfectly with savory chicken in this easy dish. Not only is mango a sweet addition, but it is packed with vitamin C, making it great for keeping skin healthy, strengthening an immune system, and helping with iron absorption. This chicken is also delicious with Kiwi Green Salsa (page 161).

FOR THE CHICKEN

Canola oil cooking spray

2 boneless, skinless chicken breasts (about ½ pound)

2 tablespoons canola oil

1 garlic clove, minced

½ teaspoon paprika

Pinch kosher salt

Pinch cayenne pepper (optional)

FOR THE MANGO SALSA

¾ cup diced ripe mango or thawed frozen mango chunks

¼ cup chopped green bell pepper

2 scallions, chopped

2 tablespoons chopped red onion

1 garlic clove, minced

1 jalapeño pepper, thinly sliced

2 tablespoons canola oil

½ teaspoon kosher salt

⅛ teaspoon ground cumin

1. Preheat the oven to 425°F. Line a rimmed baking sheet with aluminum foil or parchment paper and spritz with canola oil cooking spray.

2. Place the chicken on the prepared baking sheet. Drizzle with the oil, then sprinkle with the garlic, paprika, salt, and cayenne (if using). Roast for 20 to 25 minutes, until the chicken is cooked through.

3. While the chicken is cooking, combine all the salsa ingredients in a medium bowl and toss to mix well.

4. Serve the chicken topped with the salsa.

STORAGE: If you are sensitive to histamines or completing the elimination phase, allow leftovers to cool for at least 10 minutes, then store them in an airtight container in the freezer for up to 4 months. When you are ready to enjoy leftovers, thaw and reheat to an internal temperature of 165°F. If you are not sensitive to histamines, store leftovers in an airtight container in the refrigerator for up to 4 days.

PER SERVING: Calories: 418; Total fat: 31g; Total carbs: 15g; Fiber: 2g; Sugar: 10g; Protein: 24g; Sodium: 844mg

Chicken Skewers with Bas ͽ

PREP TIME: 10 MINUTES | COOK TIME: 15 MINUTES | YIELD: 4 SE

Bright, fresh, homemade pesto is the perfect sauce for chicken co͜
It's a dish that can be grilled in the summer when the weather is w͙
the oven when you are craving the bright, sunny summer season. You'll need metal
or wooden skewers for this.

1 cup packed fresh basil leaves

1 garlic clove, peeled

1 tablespoon shelled unsalted
sunflower seeds (if you can find
only salted, make sure there are no
other ingredients that may cause a
reaction, and adjust the salt as
needed in the recipe)

1 tablespoon hemp seeds

3½ tablespoons canola oil

¼ teaspoon kosher salt

1 pound boneless, skinless chicken
breast, cut into bite-size pieces

1. Preheat the oven to 400°F. Line a
rimmed baking sheet with parchment
paper or aluminum foil. Set a wire rack
on the baking sheet and spritz with
cooking spray. Soak skewers in water
before assembling and baking.

2. To make the pesto, pulse the basil and
garlic in a food processor until finely
chopped. Add the sunflower and hemp
seeds, pulsing to combine and scraping
down the sides as necessary. With the
machine running, slowly pour the oil
through the feed tube, add the salt, and
process until smooth and thickened.

3. Toss the chicken and 2 tablespoons
of the pesto in a large bowl until the
pieces are completed coated with the
pesto. Skewer the pieces and set the
full skewers on the rack.

4. Bake for about 15 minutes, until the
chicken is cooked through. Serve
with the remaining pesto on the side
for dipping.

> **CONTINUED ON NEXT PAGE**

Chicken Skewers with Basil Pesto

> CONTINUED

STORAGE: If you are sensitive to histamines or completing the elimination phase, allow leftovers to cool for at least 10 minutes, then store them in an airtight container in the freezer for up to 4 months. When you are ready to enjoy leftovers, thaw and reheat to an internal temperature of 165°F. If you are not sensitive to histamines, store leftovers in an airtight container in the refrigerator for up to 4 days.

ROASTED RED PEPPER PESTO VARIATION: Seed and chop ½ red bell pepper and toss with ½ teaspoon canola oil and a pinch of kosher salt. Spread out on a parchment-lined baking sheet and roast at 400°F for 20 to 25 minutes, until soft. Remove from the oven and allow to cool for about 10 minutes. Then pulse with the basil and garlic in step 2 and continue as directed above.

PER SERVING: Calories: 250; Total fat: 17g; Total carbs: 2g; Fiber: 1g; Sugar: 0g; Protein: 25g; Sodium: 326mg

Back Pocket Stir-Fry
with Rice Noodles

PREP TIME: 20 MINUTES | COOK TIME: 25 MINUTES | YIELD: 4 SERVINGS

This dish is a little sweet and subtly spicy. I call it "back pocket" because I want you to think of this more as a method rather than a specific recipe, so you can use any leftover vegetables you have on hand! This will quickly be added to your weekly rotation.

FOR THE CHICKEN AND NOODLES

1 pound boneless, skinless chicken breast, cut into bite-size pieces
1 teaspoon canola oil
¼ teaspoon kosher salt
¼ teaspoon ground black pepper
1 small garlic clove, minced or grated
½ (14-ounce) box rice noodles

FOR THE SAUCE

⅓ cup water
3 tablespoons canola oil
2 tablespoons maple syrup or agave syrup
1 tablespoon finely chopped fresh chives
1 tablespoon minced or grated peeled fresh ginger
½ teaspoon kosher salt
¼ to ½ teaspoon red pepper flakes

FOR THE STIR-FRY

2 teaspoons canola oil
3 to 4 cups chopped vegetables (a combo I like is 8 to 10 asparagus spears, 1 carrot, and 1 medium zucchini)
2 garlic cloves, minced

1. Preheat the oven to 425°F. Line a rimmed baking sheet with parchment paper or a silicone baking mat.

2. In a large bowl, toss the chicken with the oil, salt, black pepper, and garlic. Arrange in a single layer on the prepared baking sheet and bake for about 15 minutes, until cooked through.

3. While the chicken is in the oven, prepare the noodles according to the package directions. Typically, this requires soaking them in boiling water to soften. Drain.

4. Whisk the sauce ingredients together in a small bowl until smooth.

> **CONTINUED ON NEXT PAGE**

Back Pocket Stir-Fry with Rice Noodles

> CONTINUED

5. To make the stir-fry, heat the oil in a large nonstick skillet over medium-high heat. Add the chopped vegetables and garlic and cook for 5 to 8 minutes, stirring occasionally, until crisp and slightly brown.

6. Add the drained cooked noodles to the pan along with most of the sauce, reserving some for when you add the chicken. Stir to heat through and combine. Add the cooked chicken and remaining sauce, stir to combine, and serve.

STORAGE: If you are sensitive to histamines or completing the elimination phase, allow leftovers to cool for at least 10 minutes, then store them in an airtight container in the freezer for up to 4 months. When you are ready to enjoy leftovers, thaw and reheat to an internal temperature of 165°F. If you are not sensitive to histamines, store leftovers in an airtight container in the refrigerator for up to 4 days.

MAKE IT MEATLESS: You can omit the meat in this dish, and, if you are not allergic or sensitive to soy products, you can replace the chicken with tofu or tempeh after completing the elimination phase.

PER SERVING: Calories: 483; Total fat: 17g; Total carbs: 56g; Fiber: 2g; Sugar: 11g; Protein: 28g; Sodium: 652mg

Paprika Drumsticks

PREP TIME: 5 MINUTES | COOK TIME: 55 MINUTES | YIELD: 4 SERVINGS

Paprika Drumsticks are extremely easy to make—simply toss the chicken with oil and seasonings and bake. The vibrant red from the paprika gives this main dish a beautiful pop of color. I like to serve the drumsticks with Roasted Turnips with Kale and White Beans (page 153).

4 chicken drumsticks

2 teaspoons canola oil

1 garlic clove, minced or grated

1 tablespoon paprika

¼ teaspoon kosher salt

¼ teaspoon ground black pepper

1. Preheat the oven to 375°F. Line a rimmed baking sheet with parchment paper or a silicone baking mat.

2. Put the drumsticks in a large bowl and toss with the oil, garlic, paprika, salt, and pepper until well coated. Arrange on the prepared baking sheet and bake for about 30 minutes. Flip the chicken and roast for another 25 minutes, until no longer pink at the bone.

STORAGE: If you are sensitive to histamines or completing the elimination phase, allow leftovers to cool for at least 10 minutes, then store them in an airtight container in the freezer for up to 4 months. When you are ready to enjoy leftovers, thaw and reheat to an internal temperature of 165°F. If you are not sensitive to histamines, store leftovers in an airtight container in the refrigerator for up to 4 days.

PER SERVING: Calories: 138; Total fat: 12g; Total carbs: 1g; Fiber: 1g; Sugar: 0g; Protein: 16g; Sodium: 198mg

zer Chicken Meatballs

...ntastic to have on hand because you can make them when you ...spare time, then store them in the freezer for when life gets a little too ...ntic. The flax adds healthy fat and fiber, which gives these meatballs a little more staying power and a boost of nutrition. Serve them with Pesto Zucchini Noodles (page 160).

1 pound ground chicken or turkey

¼ cup ground flax meal

3 to 4 tablespoons finely chopped fresh basil

1 tablespoon chopped fresh chives

1 teaspoon kosher salt

½ teaspoon ground black pepper

½ teaspoon red pepper flakes (optional)

STORAGE: If you are sensitive to histamines or completing the elimination phase, allow leftovers to cool for at least 10 minutes, then store them in an airtight container in the freezer for up to 4 months. When you are ready to enjoy leftovers, thaw and reheat to an internal temperature of 165°F. If you are not sensitive to histamines, store leftovers in an airtight container in the refrigerator for up to 4 days.

PER SERVING: Calories: 231; Total fat: 14g; Total carbs: 3g; Fiber: 2g; Sugar: 0g; Protein: 23g; Sodium: 671mg

1. Preheat the oven to 350°F. Line a rimmed baking sheet with parchment paper or a silicone baking mat.

2. Combine the chicken or turkey, flax meal, basil, chives, salt, black pepper, and red pepper flakes in a large bowl. (You may want to use your hands here; lightly spritz them with cooking spray to prevent the mixture from sticking.) Form 16 meatballs about the size of golf balls. Place the meatballs on the prepared baking sheet and bake for 15 to 20 minutes, until cooked through.

Italian Chicken Burgers with Roasted Vegetables

PREP TIME: 20 MINUTES | COOK TIME: 20 MINUTES | YIELD: 4 SERVINGS

These zesty burgers are a favorite in my house! The roasted bell peppers and zucchini are a great way to get extra veggies in, and their delicious, naturally sweet taste is perfect with the burgers. Serve with a side of Garlic-Roasted Broccoli (page 154).

FOR THE ROASTED VEGETABLES

2 bell peppers, seeded and cut into thin strips
1 zucchini, thinly sliced
1 tablespoon canola oil
Pinch kosher salt
Pinch ground black pepper

FOR THE BURGERS

1 pound ground chicken
1½ teaspoons dried basil
1½ teaspoons dried oregano
1 teaspoon dried or chopped fresh chives
¼ teaspoon kosher salt
¼ teaspoon ground black pepper
¼ teaspoon red pepper flakes
Canola oil cooking spray
4 large cabbage leaves, for serving

1. Preheat the oven to 400°F. Line a rimmed baking sheet with parchment paper or a silicone baking mat.

2. In a large bowl, toss the bell peppers and zucchini with the oil, salt, and black pepper until well coated. Spread out in a single layer on the prepared baking sheet and roast for about 20 minutes, until tender and browned.

3. While the vegetables are roasting, combine the ground chicken with the herbs and spices. (You may want to use your hands to do this; lightly spritz them with cooking spray to prevent the mixture from sticking.) Form 4 even patties.

4. Spritz a large nonstick skillet with cooking spray and place over medium heat. When hot, add the patties to the skillet. Cook for about 6 minutes per side, until nicely browned and cooked through.

> **CONTINUED ON NEXT PAGE**

Italian Chicken Burgers with Roasted Vegetables

> CONTINUED

5. Set each burger on a cabbage leaf, top with the roasted peppers and zucchini, and serve.

STORAGE: If you are sensitive to histamines or completing the elimination phase, allow leftovers to cool for at least 10 minutes, then store them in an airtight container in the freezer for up to 4 months. When you are ready to enjoy leftovers, thaw and reheat to an internal temperature of 165°F. If you are not sensitive to histamines, store leftovers in an airtight container in the refrigerator for up to 4 days.

PER SERVING: Calories: 265; Total fat: 16g; Total carbs: 8g; Fiber: 3g; Sugar: 3g; Protein: 23g; Sodium: 285mg

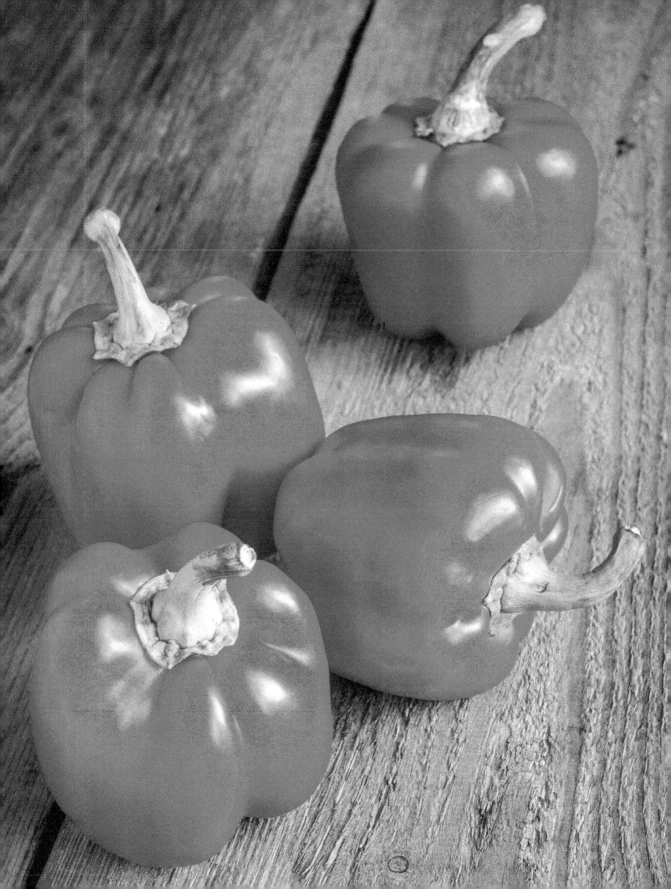

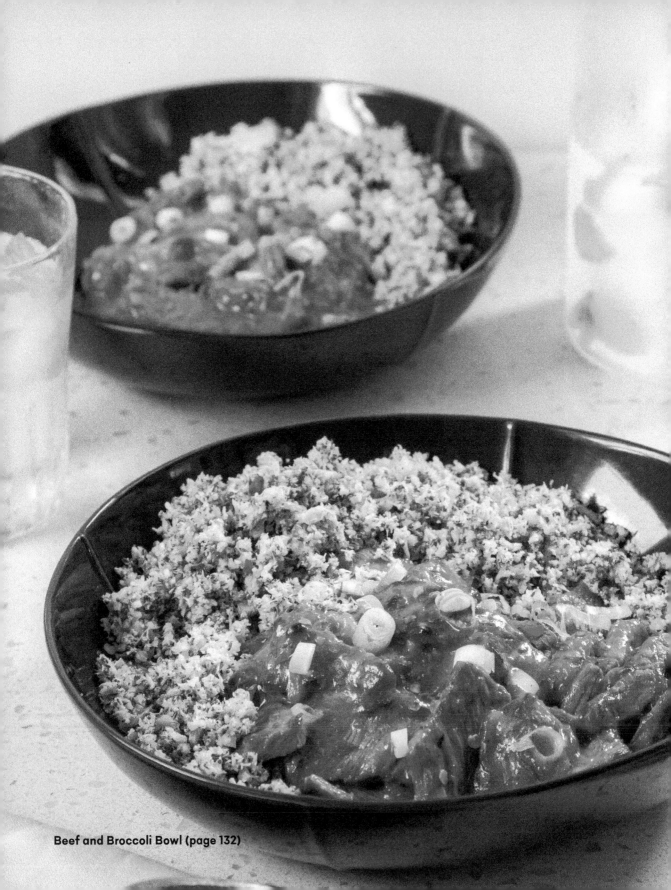

Beef and Broccoli Bowl (page 132)

CHAPTER 10

Meat

nd Broccoli Bowl

| COOK TIME: 5 MINUTES | YIELD: 4 SERVINGS

his has all the flavors of your favorite Chinese
with ingredients that will make you feel amazing

Allergy-Free Broth (page 96)

¼ cup water

3 tablespoons maple syrup or
agave syrup

1 tablespoon canola oil

2 teaspoons minced or grated peeled
fresh ginger

1 teaspoon minced garlic

1 teaspoon kosher salt

FOR THE BOWLS

1 pound boneless beef sirloin,
thinly sliced

1 teaspoon plus 1 tablespoon canola
oil, divided

1 teaspoon plus ¼ cup potato
starch, divided

1 head broccoli

1 tablespoon Allergy-Free Broth
(page 96) or water

¼ teaspoon kosher salt

⅛ teaspoon ground black pepper

2 scallions, thinly sliced

1 teaspoon red pepper flakes
(optional)

1. Whisk all the sauce ingredients
together in a small bowl. Set aside.

2. In a large bowl, toss the beef with
1 teaspoon of oil and 1 teaspoon of
potato starch until coated. Set aside to
marinate for about 10 minutes while
you prepare the broccoli.

3. While the beef is marinating, cut the
broccoli into large pieces. Working in
batches, pulse the broccoli in a food
processor until it has the texture of
rice. Transfer the broccoli rice to a
large microwave-safe bowl. Add the
broth, salt, and black pepper. Cover
lightly with a paper towel or wax
paper and steam for 45 seconds in
the microwave.

4. Remove the beef from the marinade
(reserve the marinade) and transfer to
a clean bowl. Toss with the remaining
¼ cup of potato starch.

5. Heat the remaining 1 tablespoon of
oil in a large nonstick skillet over high
heat. Add the beef; stand back to avoid
splatters. Cook for about 1 minute per
side, until browned. Transfer to a paper
towel-lined plate. Drain the excess oil
from the pan.

6. Add the reserved marinade to the pan and cook for about 1 minute, stirring, until it begins to thicken and brown. Return the beef to the pan. Reduce the heat to medium-low and cook for about another minute, stirring to coat with the sauce. Remove from the heat.

7. Divide the broccoli rice into 4 bowls, add the beef, and drizzle the sauce from the pan on top. Sprinkle with the scallions and red pepper flakes (if using) and serve.

STORAGE: If you are sensitive to histamines or completing the elimination phase, allow leftovers to cool for at least 10 minutes, then store them in an airtight container in the freezer for up to 4 months. When you are ready to enjoy leftovers, thaw and reheat to an internal temperature of 165°F. If you are not sensitive to histamines, store leftovers in an airtight container in the refrigerator for up to 4 days.

PER SERVING: Calories: 160; Total fat: 7g; Total carbs: 19g; Fiber: 14g; Sugar: 4g; Protein: 6g; Sodium: 68mg

Bunless Burger with Pesto Sauce and Dill Oven Fries

PREP TIME: 15 MINUTES | COOK TIME: 25 MINUTES | YIELD: 4 SERVINGS

The classic combination of burger and fries gets a makeover using brightly flavored dill and a fresh, homemade pesto sauce for dipping. If you time it right, the fries and burgers should finish at the same time.

FOR THE FRIES

2 russet potatoes, scrubbed and cut into ¼-inch-thick matchsticks
1 tablespoon chopped fresh dill
2 teaspoons canola oil
½ teaspoon kosher salt

FOR THE BURGERS

1 teaspoon canola oil
¼ onion, finely chopped
1 garlic clove, minced
1 pound ground beef (90% lean)
¾ teaspoon kosher salt, plus extra for sprinkling on the burgers
½ teaspoon ground black pepper
4 large cabbage leaves, for serving

FOR THE PESTO SAUCE

¼ cup water
2 tablespoons Basil Pesto (page 121)
1 small garlic clove, minced

1. Preheat the oven to 400°F. Line 2 rimmed baking sheets with parchment paper or silicone baking mats.

2. Pat the potato matchsticks dry with paper towels. In a large bowl, toss the potatoes, dill, oil, and salt together until well mixed. Arrange in a single layer on one of the prepared baking sheets. Bake for about 25 minutes, until golden brown and crisp on the outside.

3. While the fries bake, make the burgers. Heat the oil in a small skillet over medium heat. Add the onion and garlic and cook for about 5 minutes, stirring, until softened.

4. Put the ground beef in a large bowl, add the sautéed onion and garlic, salt, and pepper, and combine well. Shape the mixture into 4 even patties and place on the other prepared baking sheet. Sprinkle each patty with a pinch of salt and bake for 15 to 20 minutes, until they reach your desired degree of doneness.

5. While the fries and burgers are baking, whisk together all the pesto sauce ingredients in a small bowl until smooth.

6. Set each burger on a cabbage leaf, top with a dollop of pesto sauce, and serve with the fries.

STORAGE: If you are sensitive to histamines or completing the elimination phase, allow the beef to cool for at least 10 minutes, then store it in an airtight container in the freezer for up to 4 months. When you are ready to enjoy leftovers, thaw and reheat to an internal temperature of 165°F. If you are not sensitive to histamines, store leftover burgers in an airtight container in the refrigerator for up to 4 days.

PER SERVING: Calories: 358; Total fat: 21g; Total carbs: 16g; Fiber: 2g; Sugar: 2g; Protein: 26g; Sodium: 876mg

Spaghetti Squash and Meatballs

PREP TIME: 15 MINUTES | COOK TIME: 1 HOUR | YIELD: 4 SERVINGS

Spaghetti squash is a cousin to pumpkin in the winter squash family. Cutting one of these tough squashes in half can seem a little intimidating, so I use a method that requires cutting the squash after it is already cooked and soft. Top the spaghetti squash with my garlic sauce and meatballs for a creamy take on classic spaghetti and meatballs.

FOR THE SPAGHETTI SQUASH AND MEATBALLS

1 small spaghetti squash

1 teaspoon canola oil

½ medium onion, chopped

½ medium bell pepper (any color), seeded and chopped

1 garlic clove, minced

1 pound ground beef (90% lean)

½ cup rolled oats (certified gluten-free), ground in a food processor to a flour-like texture

1 tablespoon dried oregano

¾ teaspoon kosher salt

½ teaspoon ground black pepper

FOR THE GARLIC-HERB SAUCE

1 cup loosely packed fresh basil leaves

½ cup loosely packed fresh chives

¾ teaspoon kosher salt

2 garlic cloves, peeled

3 tablespoons hemp seeds

6 tablespoons canola oil

½ cup water

1. Preheat the oven to 400°F. Line two rimmed baking sheets with parchment paper or a silicone baking mat.

2. Use a fork to poke holes in the spaghetti squash and roast on a prepared baking sheet for about 1 hour, until soft.

3. While the squash is cooking, prepare the meatballs. Heat the oil in a small skillet over medium heat. Add the onion and bell pepper and cook for about 5 minutes, stirring occasionally, until softened. Add the garlic and cook for 30 seconds. Transfer to a large bowl and add the ground beef, oat flour, oregano, salt, and pepper. Use your hands to combine the ingredients well.

4. Roll the mixture into 16 meatballs the size of golf balls and place on the other prepared baking sheet. Bake for about 15 minutes, until cooked through. (Try to time it so they are done when the spaghetti squash is done.)

5. To make the garlic-herb sauce, pulse the basil, chives, garlic, and salt together in a food processor until finely chopped. Add the hemp seeds and pulse until finely chopped and mixed. With the machine running, slowly pour the oil through the feed tube and process until thickened. Stop the food processor and scrape down the sides as necessary. Add 1 tablespoon of water at a time to thin to your preferred consistency.

6. Once the spaghetti squash is cooked, use a hot mitt on one hand to hold the squash in place and cut the squash in half with a sharp knife in the other hand. Cool for about 5 minutes, then scoop out the seeds with a large spoon. Take a fork and rake it across the insides of each half to loosen the "spaghetti" strands. Divide them between 4 shallow bowls. Divide the sauce between the bowls and toss to coat the strands with it. Add 4 meatballs to each bowl and serve.

STORAGE: If you are sensitive to histamines or completing the elimination phase, allow the meatballs to cool for at least 10 minutes, then store them in an airtight container in the freezer for up to 4 months. When you are ready to enjoy leftovers, thaw and reheat to an internal temperature of 165°F. If you are not sensitive to histamines, store the spaghetti squash, meatballs, and sauce in separate airtight containers in the refrigerator for up to 4 days.

PER SERVING: Calories: 528; Total fat: 37g; Total carbs: 22g; Fiber: 5g; Sugar: 6g; Protein: 29g; Sodium: 972mg

Stuffed Bell Peppers

PREP TIME: 10 MINUTES | COOK TIME: 1 HOUR 40 MINUTES | YIELD: 4 SERVINGS

Stuffed peppers are one of my favorite meals when the temperatures drop. I love using the peppers as a vibrant, edible cup for the main portion of the meal—the filling.

FOR THE PEPPERS

4 bell peppers (any color)
1 teaspoon canola oil
½ teaspoon kosher salt
⅛ teaspoon ground black pepper

FOR THE FILLING

2 teaspoons canola oil
1 small onion, chopped
1 garlic clove, chopped
½ pound ground beef (90% lean)
2 teaspoons dried oregano
½ teaspoon ground cumin
1 cup Allergy-Free Broth (page 96)
½ cup brown rice
½ teaspoon kosher salt
⅛ teaspoon ground black pepper
½ (15-ounce) can white beans, rinse and drained
1 tablespoon fresh oregano

1. Preheat the oven to 400°F.
2. Cut the top off each pepper and reserve. Scrape the seeds out of the inside of each pepper, then rub the outsides with the oil and sprinkle with the salt and pepper. Set aside.
3. To make the filling, heat the oil in a large nonstick skillet over medium heat. Add the onion and garlic and cook for 2 to 3 minutes, stirring occasionally, until softened and translucent. Add the ground beef, dried oregano, and cumin. Stir and cook for about 5 minutes, until no longer pink. Add the broth and rice and stir to combine. Cover, reduce the heat to low, and simmer for about 30 minutes, until the liquid is absorbed. Season with the salt and pepper, then mix in the beans.

4. Divide the filling among the 4 peppers and place the pepper tops back on. Set the peppers in a baking dish that allows them to stand upright. Cover the dish with aluminum foil and bake for about 1 hour, until the peppers are tender and the filling is hot.

5. Sprinkle with the fresh oregano and serve.

STORAGE: If you are sensitive to histamines or completing the elimination phase, do not consume leftovers of this dish, as it does not freeze well. If you are not sensitive to histamines, store leftovers in an airtight container in the refrigerator for up to 4 days.

PER SERVING: Calories: 308; Total fat: 10g; Total carbs: 39g; Fiber: 5g; Sugar: 1g; Protein: 18g; Sodium: 768mg

Taco-Stuffed Sweet Potatoes

PREP TIME: 10 MINUTES | COOK TIME: 1 HOUR | YIELD: 2 SERVINGS

Sweet potatoes are a nutrient-dense base (rich in fiber and vitamin A) for fajita veggies and taco meat. While an hour may seem like a long time to cook a sweet potato, this method allows all the natural sugars to come out and gives the sweet potatoes an out-of-this-world flavor.

2 medium sweet potatoes

FOR THE FAJITA VEGETABLES

½ bell pepper, seeded and cut into thin strips

½ zucchini, thinly sliced

½ onion, thinly sliced

2 teaspoons canola oil

2 teaspoons ground cumin

½ teaspoon dried oregano

¼ teaspoon kosher salt

FOR THE GROUND BEEF

½ pound ground beef (90% lean)

1 teaspoon ground cumin

1 teaspoon paprika

½ teaspoon kosher salt

⅛ teaspoon ground black pepper

1. Preheat the oven to 425°F. Line a rimmed baking sheet with parchment paper or a silicone baking mat.

2. Pierce the sweet potatoes several times with a fork. Wrap in aluminum foil and place directly on the oven rack; bake for about 1 hour, until tender.

3. While the sweet potatoes are baking, in a large bowl, toss the fajita vegetables with the oil, cumin, oregano, and salt. Arrange in a single layer on the prepared baking sheet and roast for about 25 minutes, until tender and browned. Try to time it so the sweet potatoes and vegetables finish at the same time.

4. While the potatoes and vegetables are cooking, brown the ground beef in a nonstick skillet with the cumin, paprika, salt, and pepper. Stir constantly for 5 to 8 minutes, until cooked through. Cover and remove from the heat.

5. Cut the cooked sweet potatoes in half, top with the browned beef and fajita vegetables, and serve.

STORAGE: If you are sensitive to histamines or completing the elimination phase, do not consume leftovers of this dish, as it does not freeze well. If you are not sensitive to histamines, store leftovers in an airtight container in the refrigerator for up to 4 days.

PER SERVING: Calories: 397; Total fat: 15g; Total carbs: 39g; Fiber: 6g; Sugar: 8g; Protein: 27g; Sodium: 965mg

Pan-Seared S[...]

PREP TIME: 5 MINUTES | COOK TIME: 5 MINUTES | Y[...]

This recipe is about as simple as they come, but it turns o[...] steak every single time.

½ teaspoon kosher salt
⅛ teaspoon ground black pepper
1 small garlic clove, minced
2 (4-ounce) boneless steaks

1. Set a rimmed baking sheet under the broiler and preheat the broiler. Preheat a cast-iron skillet over medium-high heat.
2. Rub the salt, pepper, and garlic into both sides of the steaks.
3. Sear the steak[...] 15 seconds on e[...] to the hot bakin[...] oven. Broil for 2 minutes per side or to your desired degree of doneness.

> **STORAGE:** If you are sensitive to histamines or completing the elimination phase, do not consume leftovers of this dish, as it does not freeze well. If you are not sensitive to histamines, store leftovers in an airtight container in the refrigerator for up to 4 days.

PER SERVING: Calories: 176; Total fat: 8g; Total carbs: 0g; Fiber: 0g; Sugar: 0g; Protein: 23g; Sodium: 664mg

Egg Roll Bowls

PREP TIME: 15 MINUTES | COOK TIME: 15 MINUTES | YIELD: 4 SERVINGS

Love traditional egg rolls? Then you will love having all the flavors of your favorite Asian side dish sautéed together and tossed in a bowl with brown rice. Best of all, this mouthwatering meal comes together really quickly.

1 tablespoon canola oil

3 garlic cloves, minced

1 (1-inch) piece fresh ginger, peeled and minced or grated

1 teaspoon kosher salt

¼ teaspoon cayenne pepper

1 pound ground pork or turkey

5 to 6 cups shredded green or red cabbage

3 medium carrots, peeled and chopped

2 cups Simple Brown Rice (page 162)

½ cup chopped scallions

1. Heat the oil in a large skillet over medium heat. Add the garlic and ginger and cook for about 1 minute, stirring, until fragrant. Add the salt, cayenne, and pork. Cook and break apart the meat for 5 to 8 minutes, until it is browned.

2. Add the cabbage and carrots. Cook for about 5 minutes, gently tossing, until the vegetables are crisp-tender.

3. Serve over the rice, sprinkled with the scallions.

STORAGE: If you are sensitive to histamines or completing the elimination phase, allow leftovers to cool to room temperature, then store them in an airtight container in the freezer for up to 4 months. When you are ready to enjoy leftovers, thaw and reheat to an internal temperature of 165°F. If you are not sensitive to histamines, store leftovers in an airtight container in the refrigerator for up to 4 days.

TIME-SAVER TIP: Cook the rice ahead of time.

PER SERVING: Calories: 486; Total fat: 29g; Total carbs: 33g; Fiber: 5g; Sugar: 6g; Protein: 23g; Sodium: 696mg

Herby Pork Meatballs with Roasted Apples

PREP TIME: 10 MINUTES | COOK TIME: 20 MINUTES | YIELD: 4 SERVINGS

Apples and pork are a pair made in heaven. Roasting the apples brings out sweet flavors that perfectly complement the savory herbs in these meatballs.

1 pound ground pork or chicken

1 tablespoon chopped fresh chives

1 tablespoon chopped fresh basil

1 teaspoon red pepper flakes (optional)

½ teaspoon kosher salt

¼ teaspoon ground black pepper

1 apple, cored and diced

1. Preheat the oven to 350°F. Line a rimmed baking sheet with parchment paper or a silicone baking mat.

2. In a large bowl, combine the ground pork, chives, basil, red pepper flakes (if using), salt, and black pepper. It's easiest to use your hands to mix this up. Form 16 meatballs the size of golf balls and place on the prepared baking sheet. Scatter the apples around the meatballs. Bake for 15 to 20 minutes, until the meatballs are cooked through and the apples are tender.

STORAGE: If you are sensitive to histamines or completing the elimination phase, allow leftovers to cool to room temperature, then store them in an airtight container in the freezer for up to 4 months. When you are ready to enjoy leftovers, thaw and reheat to an internal temperature of 145°F. If you are not sensitive to histamines, store leftovers in an airtight container in the refrigerator for up to 4 days.

PER SERVING: Calories: 326; Total fat: 24g; Total carbs: 7g; Fiber: 1g; Sugar: 5g; Protein: 19g; Sodium: 354mg

...ed Pork Chops

| COOK TIME: 20 MINUTES | YIELD: 4 SERVINGS

...tly frying and then stewing. For this recipe, you'll ...wn it in a pan before reducing the apple juice and ...this subtly sweet sauce. Pair this with a vegetable ...plete!

1 teaspoon dried rubbed sage
¾ teaspoon kosher salt
¼ teaspoon ground black pepper
4 (4-ounce) boneless pork loin chops
1 tablespoon canola oil
¾ cup 100% apple juice (check the ingredient list)

1. Mix the garlic, sage, salt, and pepper together in a small bowl. Rub on both sides of the pork chops.

2. In a large nonstick skillet, heat the oil over medium-high heat. Brown the pork chops for 3 minutes on each side. Transfer them to a plate.

3. Add the apple juice to the pan and use a wooden spoon to scrape up any browned bits from the bottom of the pan. Cook for about 2 minutes, uncovered, until the juice is reduced to nearly half. Return the pork chops to the pan and bring the liquid back to a boil.

4. Cover, reduce the heat to low, and simmer for about 8 minutes, until the pork is cooked through.

5. Serve the chops with the pan sauce spooned over it.

STORAGE: If you are sensitive to histamines or completing the elimination phase, allow leftovers to cool for at least 10 minutes, then store them in an airtight container in the freezer for up to 4 months. When you are ready to enjoy leftovers, thaw and reheat to an internal temperature of 145°F. If you are not sensitive to histamines, store in an airtight container in the refrigerator for up to 4 days.

PER SERVING: Calories: 193; Total fat: 8g; Total carbs: 6g; Fiber: 0g; Sugar: 5g; Protein: 23g; Sodium: 646mg

Sautéed Pork Loin

PREP TIME: 5 MINUTES | COOK TIME: 10 MINUTES | YIELD: 4 SERVINGS

Here's a simple method for preparing pork loin that comes together in just about 10 minutes and goes perfectly with any side dish.

1 tablespoon canola oil

1 pound pork tenderloin, cut into 1-inch cubes

1/2 teaspoon kosher salt

1/8 teaspoon ground black pepper

1 garlic clove, minced

1. Heat the oil in a large nonstick skillet over medium-high heat.

2. Toss the pork with the salt, pepper, and garlic. Add to the hot skillet and cook for 10 minutes, uncovered, until cooked through, stirring occasionally.

STORAGE: If you are sensitive to histamines or completing the elimination phase, allow leftovers to cool for at least 10 minutes, then store them in an airtight container in the freezer for up to 4 months. When you are ready to enjoy leftovers, thaw and reheat to an internal temperature of 165°F. If you are not sensitive to histamines, store leftovers in the refrigerator for up to 4 days.

PER SERVING: Calories: 194; Total fat: 11g; Total carbs: 1g; Fiber: 0g; Sugar: 0g; Protein: 21g; Sodium: 692mg

Slow Cooker Pork Stir-Fry

PREP TIME: 15 MINUTES | COOK TIME: 2 TO 4 HOURS | YIELD: 4 SERVINGS

Pork cooked in the slow cooker comes out tender and full of flavor. The slow cooker does all the heavy lifting of perfectly cooking the meat, then you can chop your vegetables and sauté everything together once the pork is cooked through. Serve this on its own or over Simple Brown Rice (page 162).

1 pound pork tenderloin, trimmed of excess fat

3 tablespoons minced or grated peeled fresh ginger

2 garlic cloves, minced

2 tablespoons sunflower seed butter, divided

1 tablespoon maple syrup or agave syrup

1 teaspoon kosher salt

¼ cup water

2 teaspoons canola oil

2 medium carrots, peeled and thinly sliced on the bias

1 cup broccoli florets

1 bell pepper (any color), seeded and cut into thin strips

1 cup frozen peas

1 cup sliced scallions

¼ cup shelled unsalted sunflower seeds (if you can only find salted, make sure there are no other ingredients that may cause a reaction, and adjust the salt as needed in the recipe)

Red pepper flakes (optional)

1. Put the pork tenderloin in the slow cooker. In a small bowl, stir together the ginger, garlic, 1 tablespoon of sunflower seed butter, maple syrup, salt, and water. Pour into the slow cooker, spreading it with a spoon. Cover the slow cooker and cook on low for 2 to 4 hours. Transfer the pork to a large plate and let rest for 10 minutes. Skim the fat from the cooking liquid and discard. Shred the pork with two forks or cut it into bite-size pieces.

2. Heat the oil in a large nonstick skillet over medium-high heat. Add the carrots, broccoli, and bell pepper. Cook for about 7 minutes, stirring, until crisp-tender. Add the frozen peas and cook for about 2 minutes, until heated through. Transfer the vegetables to a bowl and set aside.

3. Spoon the defatted cooking liquid from the slow cooker into the skillet. Add the remaining 1 tablespoon of sunflower seed butter and whisk to combine. Add the pork, cooked vegetables, scallions, sunflower seeds, and red pepper flakes (if using). Toss to coat everything with the sauce and serve.

STORAGE: If you are sensitive to histamines or completing the elimination phase, do not consume leftovers of this dish, as it does not freeze well. If you are not sensitive to histamines, store leftovers in an airtight container in the refrigerator for up to 4 days.

PER SERVING: Calories: 425; Total fat: 20g; Total carbs: 21g; Fiber: 6g; Sugar: 9g; Protein: 40g; Sodium: 747mg

Greek Meatball Salad

PREP TIME: 15 MINUTES | COOK TIME: 5 MINUTES | YIELD: 4 SERVINGS

Lamb is a source of many vitamins and minerals such as vitamin B12, iron, and zinc. I like to broil these mini-meatballs to save a ton of time but maintain all the flavor. Pop these meatballs on a bed of fresh vegetables and dress them with this creamy green dressing and your meal is ready to go.

FOR THE MEATBALLS

Canola oil cooking spray

1 pound ground lamb or turkey

1/2 red onion, finely chopped

1 tablespoon minced fresh oregano

1 small garlic clove, minced

1/2 teaspoon kosher salt

FOR THE DRESSING

1/2 cup loosely packed fresh chives

1/2 cup fresh oregano leaves

2 garlic cloves, peeled

3 tablespoons hemp seeds

1/2 teaspoon kosher salt

6 tablespoons canola oil

1/2 cup water

FOR THE SALAD

6 cups baby kale

1/2 bell pepper (any color), seeded and cut into thin strips

1/2 cucumber, chopped

1. Preheat the broiler. Line a rimmed baking sheet with aluminum foil. Spritz with canola oil cooking spray.

2. In a large bowl, combine the ground lamb, onion, oregano, garlic, and salt thoroughly. Roll into 24 meatballs and arrange in a single layer on the prepared baking sheet. Broil for about 5 minutes, until cooked through, turning them once for even browning.

3. For the dressing, pulse the chives, oregano, and garlic in a food processor until finely chopped. Add the hemp seeds and salt and pulse until finely chopped and mixed. With the machine running, slowly pour the oil through the feed tube and process until thickened. Stop the food processor and scrape down the sides as necessary. Add 1 tablespoon of water at a time to thin to the consistency you prefer.

4. To assemble the salads, divide the kale, bell pepper, and cucumber into 4 bowls, dollop the dressing on top, and toss to coat well. Top each salad with 6 meatballs and serve.

> **STORAGE:** If you are sensitive to histamines or completing the elimination phase, allow leftover meatballs to cool for at least 10 minutes, then store them in an airtight container in the freezer for up to 4 months. When you are ready to enjoy leftovers, thaw and reheat to an internal temperature of 165°F. If you are not sensitive to histamines, store leftover meatballs, salad, and dressing in separate containers in the refrigerator for up to 4 days.

PER SERVING: Calories: 578; Total fat: 51g; Total carbs: 5g; Fiber: 3g; Sugar: 2g; Protein: 23g; Sodium: 672mg

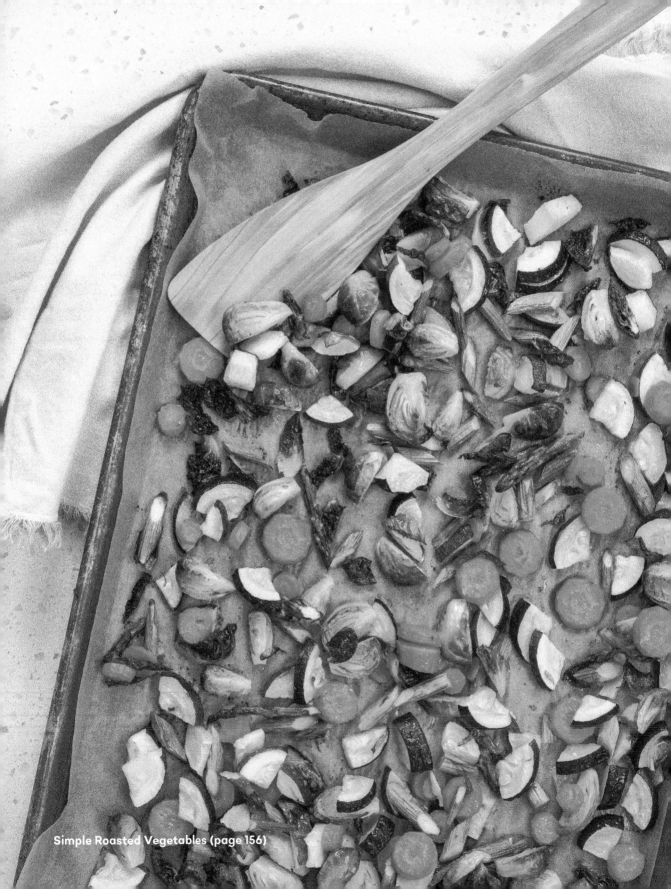

Simple Roasted Vegetables (page 156)

CHAPTER 11

Easy Sides

Dilled Bean Salad with Carrots and Quinoa

PREP TIME: 10 MINUTES | COOK TIME: 15 MINUTES | YIELD: 4 SERVINGS

I love that this dish has protein from both quinoa and beans. Enjoying a larger portion of this salad could definitely serve as the main part of your meal. This dish is great to make at the end of the week with any leftover beans, quinoa, carrots, or onions you cooked for recipes at the start of the week.

2 medium carrots, peeled and diced

¼ cup sliced onion

2 tablespoons plus 1 teaspoon canola oil

½ teaspoon kosher salt, divided

1 cup Perfectly Cooked Quinoa (page 163)

1 cup canned beans (any kind), rinsed and drained

3 tablespoons chopped fresh dill

1 garlic clove, minced

⅛ teaspoon ground black pepper

1. Preheat the oven to 400°F. Line a rimmed baking sheet with parchment paper or a silicone baking mat.

2. Toss the carrots and onion with 1 teaspoon of oil and a pinch of salt. Spread them out in a single layer on the prepared baking sheet and roast for about 15 minutes, until tender.

3. Combine the quinoa, roasted vegetables, and beans in a large bowl. Stir to combine.

4. In a small bowl, combine the dill, garlic, remaining 2 tablespoons of oil, remaining salt, and pepper. Pour over the quinoa and carrot mixture and stir to combine. Cover and set aside for about 30 minutes to allow the flavors to meld, then serve.

STORAGE: Store in an airtight container in the refrigerator for up to 4 days.

PER SERVING: Calories: 200; Total fat: 9g; Total carbs: 24g; Fiber: 5g; Sugar: 2g; Protein: 6g; Sodium: 217mg

Roasted Turnips with Kale and White Beans

PREP TIME: 10 MINUTES | COOK TIME: 30 MINUTES | YIELD: 4 SERVINGS

Turnips are part of the cruciferous vegetable family like cabbage, cauliflower, and broccoli. Cruciferous vegetables are packed with vitamins, minerals, fiber, and natural cancer-fighting properties. Preparing turnips may be something new for you, but their crunchy texture and neutral-earthy flavor make it easy to reap the rewards of this root vegetable.

FOR THE TURNIPS

- 2 medium turnips, peeled and cut into bite-size pieces
- 2 teaspoons canola oil
- ¼ teaspoon kosher salt
- ¼ teaspoon ground black pepper
- ¼ teaspoon paprika

FOR THE KALE AND WHITE BEANS

- 3 tablespoons canola oil
- 3 tablespoons water
- 1 garlic clove, minced
- ¾ teaspoon kosher salt
- ¼ teaspoon paprika
- 3 cups loosely packed baby kale
- 1 (15-ounce) can white beans, rinsed and drained
- ⅓ cup shelled unsalted sunflower seeds (if you can find only salted, make sure there are no other ingredients that may cause a reaction, and adjust the salt as needed in the recipe)

1. Preheat the oven to 400°F. Line a rimmed baking sheet with parchment paper or a silicone baking mat.
2. Toss the turnips with the oil, salt, pepper, and paprika. Spread in a single layer on the prepared baking sheet and roast for 25 to 30 minutes, until crisp on the outside and slightly tender on the inside. Remove from the oven and allow to cool slightly.
3. In a large bowl, whisk together the oil, water, garlic, salt, and paprika. Add the kale, beans, sunflower seeds, and turnips and toss to combine. The mixture is a tasty combination of cold and warm.

STORAGE: You can store leftovers in an airtight container in the refrigerator for up to 4 days, but this dish is best served fresh.

PER SERVING: Calories: 282; Total fat: 18g; Total carbs: 22g; Fiber: 7g; Sugar: 4g; Protein: 8g; Sodium: 636mg

Garlic-Roasted Broccoli

PREP TIME: 5 MINUTES | COOK TIME: 30 MINUTES | YIELD: 2 TO 4 SERVINGS

I predict that this simple side dish will become a regular mealtime addition for you. I make roasted vegetables often because I can't get enough of the crunchy outside and soft inside texture.

1 head broccoli, cut into florets

2 teaspoons canola oil

½ teaspoon kosher salt

1 garlic clove, minced

1. Preheat the oven to 400°F. Line a rimmed baking sheet with parchment paper or a silicone baking mat.

2. In a medium bowl, toss the broccoli with the oil, salt, and garlic. Spread the broccoli in a single layer on the prepared baking sheet and roast for about 30 minutes, until slightly crisp on the outside.

PER SERVING (WHEN SERVES 2): Calories: 127; Total fat: 6g; Total carbs: 16g; Fiber: 9g; Sugar: 5g; Protein: 9g; Sodium: 664mg

Mediterranean Roasted Asparag

PREP TIME: 10 MINUTES | COOK TIME: 25 MINUTES | YIE

In this easy recipe, simple asparagus gets dressed up with
Adding lots of herbs and spices is a great way to transform a food you ejy
into something brand new.

½ pound asparagus, trimmed

¼ cup thinly sliced red onion

6 garlic cloves, minced

1 tablespoon canola oil

½ teaspoon dried oregano

½ teaspoon kosher salt

⅛ teaspoon ground black pepper

¼ cup chopped fresh dill

1. Preheat the oven to 400°F. Line a rimmed baking sheet with parchment paper or a silicone baking mat.

2. Put the asparagus, onion, and garlic on the prepared baking sheet. Drizzle with the oil and sprinkle with the oregano, salt, and pepper. Toss to coat, then spread out in a single layer. Roast for 20 to 25 minutes, until crisp and slightly browned.

3. Toss the roasted asparagus with the dill and serve.

PER SERVING: Calories: 56; Total fat: 4g; Total carbs: 5g; Fiber: 2g; Sugar: 2g; Protein: 2g; Sodium: 293mg

Simple Roasted Vegetables

PREP TIME: 10 MINUTES | COOK TIME: 30 MINUTES | YIELD: 4 SERVINGS

This recipe is sort of a "choose your own adventure" side dish. I'm offering one of my favorite combinations here, but you can use any you like, so long as they are on the list of vegetables to enjoy while you are completing the elimination phase (see page 29). You'll need about 6 cups of chopped vegetables total.

**10 Brussels sprouts, halved
or quartered**

**10 asparagus spears, trimmed
and sliced**

4 small carrots, peeled and chopped

1 small zucchini, chopped

1 tablespoon canola oil

½ teaspoon kosher salt

1. Preheat the oven to 400°F. Line a rimmed baking sheet with parchment paper or a silicone baking mat.

2. In a large bowl, toss the Brussels sprouts, asparagus, carrots, and zucchini with the oil and salt until well coated.

3. Spread the vegetables out in a single layer on the prepared baking sheet and roast for about 30 minutes, until slightly golden brown and crisp. This dish is best served freshly made.

TIME-SAVER TIP: Chop the vegetables a day in advance and store in an airtight container in the refrigerator.

PER SERVING: Calories: 86; Total fat: 4g; Total carbs: 12g; Fiber: 4g; Sugar: 5g; Protein: 3g; Sodium: 341mg

Roasted Brussels Sprouts with Wild Rice

PREP TIME: 10 MINUTES | COOK TIME: 1 HOUR | YIELD: 4 SERVINGS

The paprika and sage in this dish really make these Brussels sprouts taste like a bowl full of comfort. Brussels sprouts are a cruciferous vegetable filled with vitamin K and vitamin C and many other vitamins and minerals. Wild rice provides a chewy texture that perfectly contrasts with the crisp Brussels sprouts.

FOR THE RICE

⅓ cup wild rice, rinsed and drained
1⅓ cups water
Pinch kosher salt

FOR THE BRUSSELS SPROUTS

2 cups quartered Brussels sprouts
1 teaspoon canola oil
¼ teaspoon kosher salt

TO FINISH

1 tablespoon canola oil
1 garlic clove, minced
1 teaspoon dried rubbed sage
¼ teaspoon kosher salt
¼ teaspoon ground black pepper
⅛ teaspoon paprika
¼ cup chopped scallions

1. Preheat the oven to 400°F and line a rimmed baking sheet with parchment paper or a silicone baking mat.

2. Combine the rice and water in a medium saucepan, add the salt, and bring to a boil over high heat. Reduce the heat to low, cover, and simmer for 45 to 55 minutes, until the rice is tender but still a little chewy. Drain off any remaining liquid.

3. While the rice is cooking, in a medium bowl, toss the Brussels sprouts with the oil and salt. Arrange in a single layer on the prepared baking sheet and roast for about 25 minutes, until tender.

4. Combine the cooked wild rice and roasted Brussels sprouts in a large bowl. Add the oil, garlic, sage, salt, pepper, and paprika. Toss to combine, then sprinkle with the scallions and serve.

> **CONTINUED ON NEXT PAGE**

Roasted Brussels Sprouts with Wild Rice

> CONTINUED

STORAGE: Store in an airtight container in the refrigerator for up to 4 days. Reheat before serving.

TIME-SAVER TIP: Cook the wild rice ahead of time.

PER SERVING: Calories: 120; Total fat: 5g; Total carbs: 16g; Fiber: 3g; Sugar: 1g; Protein: 4g; Sodium: 342mg

Garlic-Ginger Bok Choy

PREP TIME: 5 MINUTES | COOK TIME: 5 MINUTES | YIELD: 4 SERVINGS

Bok choy is a variety of Chinese cabbage that has soft green leaves and a crunchy white stem. It's high in the mineral selenium, which is great for brain health, the immune system, cancer protection, and thyroid health.

2 teaspoons canola oil

1 garlic clove, minced

2 teaspoons minced or grated peeled fresh ginger

4 baby bok choy, halved lengthwise

2 tablespoons water

½ teaspoon kosher salt

1. Heat the oil in a large nonstick skillet over medium-high heat. Add the garlic and ginger and cook for about 30 seconds, stirring, until golden.

2. Add the bok choy, cut-side down. Add the water, reduce the heat to low, cover, and cook for 2 minutes.

3. Turn the bok choy cut-side up and increase the heat to medium-high. Sprinkle with the salt and cook for about 2 more minutes, until the stems are tender.

PER SERVING: Calories: 31; Total fat: 2g; Total carbs: 2g; Fiber: 1g; Sugar: 1g; Protein: 1g; Sodium: 337mg

Pesto Zucchini Noodles

PREP TIME: 5 MINUTES | COOK TIME: 2 MINUTES | YIELD: 2 SERVINGS

I'm calling this a side dish, but you could easily increase the portion size, serve it with your favorite protein, and make it into a main dish.

Canola oil cooking spray

1 medium zucchini, spiralized into noodles

2 tablespoons Basil Pesto (page 121)

¼ teaspoon kosher salt

1. Coat the bottom of a medium skillet with cooking spray and heat over medium-high heat. Add the zucchini noodles and cook for 1 to 2 minutes, stirring, to cook off some of their moisture and heat them through.

2. Remove from the heat and toss with the pesto and salt. Serve, topped with more pesto if you like.

> **TIME-SAVER TIP:** Spiralize the zucchini a day in advance.

PER SERVING: Calories: 155; Total fat: 15g; Total carbs: 5g; Fiber: 2g; Sugar: 2g; Protein: 3g; Sodium: 447mg

Kiwi Green Salsa

PREP TIME: 10 MINUTES | YIELD: 6 SERVINGS

This recipe changes up the usual red salsa for a combination of sweet, savory, and green with kiwi. This fresh and vibrant dish has lots of flavor, is not too spicy, and is perfect for sharing with a crowd. It's a tasty partner for Taco-Stuffed Sweet Potatoes (page 140) or Chicken with Chimichurri (page 113).

5 kiwis, peeled and diced

½ cup chopped green tomato

¼ cup chopped red onion

¼ cup chopped green bell pepper

2 scallions, thinly sliced

1 garlic clove, minced

1 jalapeño pepper, seeded and thinly sliced

2 tablespoons canola oil

½ teaspoon kosher salt

In a medium bowl, toss all the ingredients together until well mixed. Taste and adjust the seasoning if needed.

STORAGE: Store in an airtight container in the refrigerator for up to 7 days.

PER SERVING (¼ CUP): Calories: 90; Total fat: 5g; Total carbs: 12g; Fiber: 3g; Sugar: 7g; Protein: 1g; Sodium: 200mg

Simple Brown Rice

COOK TIME: 40 MINUTES | YIELD: 4 SERVINGS

Brown rice is a nutrient-rich whole grain that is a perfect addition to many meals, salads, and side dishes. It's high in many vitamins such as folate and B12, minerals like potassium and calcium, and antioxidants like phenols and flavonols. It's also a blank canvas for flavor, so mix in any spices or seasonings that sound good to you.

2¼ cups water or Allergy-Free Broth (page 96)

1 cup brown rice

¼ teaspoon kosher salt

Optional seasonings: ½ teaspoon cumin seeds, chopped fresh chives or scallions, minced garlic, a drizzle of olive oil, chopped fresh basil and oregano

1. Combine the water and rice in a medium saucepan. Bring to a boil over high heat. Cover, reduce the heat to low, and simmer (no peeking!) for 30 minutes.

2. Remove the pan from the heat and let steam, covered, for another 10 minutes. The water should all be evaporated at this point.

3. Fluff the rice with a fork. Season with salt and add the optional seasonings, if you like.

STORAGE: Store in an airtight container in the refrigerator for 4 days.

PER SERVING (½ CUP): Calories: 160; Total fat: 1g; Total carbs: 35g; Fiber: 2g; Sugar: 0g; Protein: 4g; Sodium: 145mg

Perfectly Cooked Quinoa

COOK TIME: 10 TO 15 MINUTES | YIELD: 6 SERVINGS

Even though we eat it like a grain, quinoa is actually a seed. It has a chewy texture and slightly nutty flavor and contains all the essential amino acids, making it a great plant protein source.

1 cup quinoa (any color)

2 cups water

¼ teaspoon kosher salt

STORAGE: Store in an airtight container in the refrigerator for up to 5 days.

1. In a medium saucepan, combine the quinoa, water, and salt. Cover and bring to a boil. Reduce the heat to low and simmer for 10 to 15 minutes, until the water is absorbed and the quinoa is done. You'll know it is ready when the germ starts to separate from the seed, with a little white curl coming off the main round part.

2. Fluff the quinoa with a fork and serve.

PER SERVING (½ CUP): Calories: 115; Total fat: 2g; Total carbs: 21g; Fiber: 2g; Sugar: 2g; Protein: 4g; Sodium: 97mg

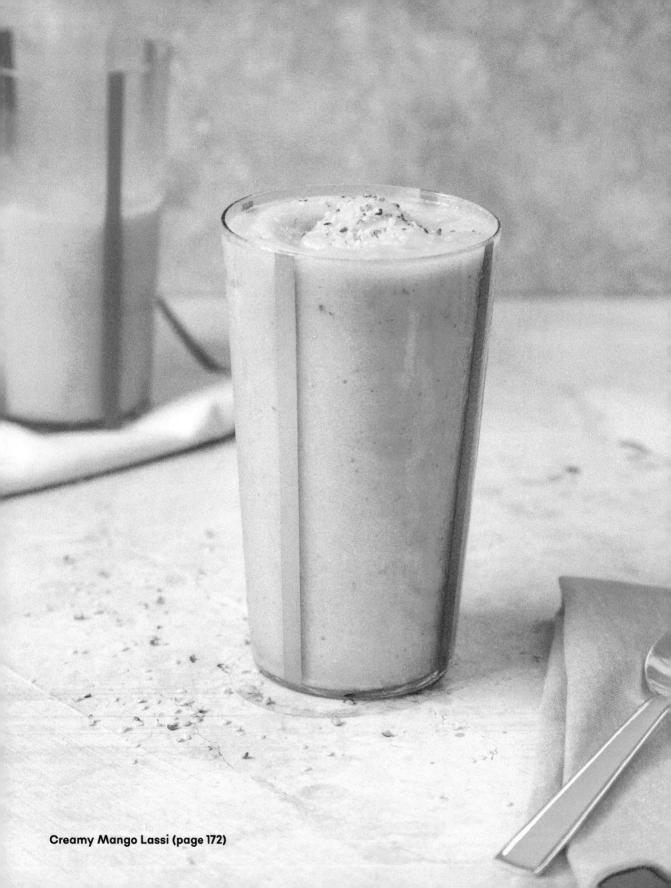

Creamy Mango Lassi (page 172)

CHAPTER 12

Sweets and Snacks

Mango-Banana Nice Cream

PREP TIME: 5 MINUTES | YIELD: 2 SERVINGS

This cool, creamy treat has the texture of soft serve and is the perfect treat for a hot summer night.

2 cups frozen mango chunks

1 frozen banana, cut into chunks

Pinch kosher salt

2/3 cup unsweetened rice, hemp, oat, or flax milk (check the ingredient list for any potential foods not allowed during the elimination phase)

1 to 2 teaspoons maple syrup (optional)

1. Combine the mango, banana, and salt in a food processor and process for just short of 1 minute, until crumbly.

2. With the machine running, slowly pour the milk and maple syrup (if using) through the feed tube and blend for 1 to 2 minutes, until very smooth and creamy, like ice cream. Stop the machine and scrape down the sides as needed. Serve immediately.

> **STORAGE:** Store in an airtight container in the freezer and scoop it out like regular ice cream for about 2 weeks.

PER SERVING: Calories: 185; Total fat: 1g; Total carbs: 47g; Fiber: 7g; Sugar: 31g; Protein: 2g; Sodium: 132mg

Oatmeal Snack Bit

PREP TIME: 10 MINUTES | YIELD: 24 BITES

Bites like these keep me going in the middle of a big project, after a hard workout. They are easy to store because they do space. Using sunflower seeds and sunflower seed butter packs these healthy fat, while the oats give it filling fiber. Noshing on a snack like this will tide you over between meals.

¾ cup rolled oats (certified gluten-free)

½ cup sunflower seed butter

2 tablespoons shelled unsalted sunflower seeds (if you can find only salted, make sure there are no other ingredients that may cause a reaction, and adjust the salt as needed in the recipe)

1 tablespoon maple syrup or agave syrup

Pinch kosher salt

1. Line a plate or small baking sheet with parchment or wax paper.
2. In a large bowl, combine the oats, sunflower seed butter, sunflower seeds, maple syrup, and salt and mix well to combine. I like to mix with my hands!
3. Roll the mixture into walnut-size balls and place on the prepared plate or baking sheet. Freeze for at least 30 minutes.
4. Allow to sit on the counter for a couple of minutes to thaw before eating.

STORAGE: Store in an airtight container in the freezer for up to 3 months.

PER SERVING (1 BITE): Calories: 49; Total fat: 3g; Total carbs: 4g; Fiber: 1g; Sugar: 1g; Protein: 2g; Sodium: 27mg

Mango Oat Crumble Bars

PREP TIME: 10 MINUTES | COOK TIME: 45 MINUTES | YIELD: 16 BARS

If you love crumb topping, you will adore these bars. The hardest part about making them is waiting for them to cool down completely after baking. If you like, substitute blueberries for the mango.

1⅓ cups rolled oats (certified gluten-free) plus 6 tablespoons rolled oats (certified gluten-free), ground in a food processor to a flour-like texture

½ cup cane sugar

¾ teaspoon minced or grated peeled fresh ginger

¼ teaspoon baking soda

¼ teaspoon kosher salt

⅓ cup canola oil

1 flax egg (see page 85)

1 cup chopped fresh or frozen mango

1 teaspoon potato starch

1. Preheat the oven to 350°F. Line an 8-by-8-inch baking pan with parchment paper with a little bit hanging over two of the sides (you will use these as "handles" later).

2. Combine the oats, oat flour, sugar, ginger, baking soda, and salt in a medium bowl. Add the oil and mix until completely combined. Scoop out ½ cup of the crumbs and set aside.

3. Mix the flax egg into the remaining crumbs. Press this mixture into the bottom of the prepared baking pan. Scatter the mango over the crumb mixture, then sprinkle with the potato starch. Sprinkle the reserved crumbs over the top of the mango (some fruit will show through).

4. Bake for 40 to 45 minutes, until the fruit is bubbling and the crumb topping is light golden brown and very aromatic. Let cool completely before cutting into 16 squares. You can place the pan in the refrigerator to speed this up.

STORAGE: Store in an airtight container in the refrigerator for up to 5 days or in the freezer for up to a month.

PER SERVING (1 BAR): Calories: 103; Total fat: 5g; Total carbs: 14g; Fiber: 1g; Sugar: 8g; Protein: 1g; Sodium: 93mg

No-Bake Sunbutter Cookies

PREP TIME: 10 MINUTES | COOK TIME: 5 MINUTES | YIELD: 12 MEDIUM COOKIES
OR 24 SMALL COOKIES

Have you ever had peanut butter and chocolate no-bake cookies? They were a favorite of mine growing up and the inspiration for this recipe. The method is similar, but this version is allergy-free.

1 cup cane sugar

¾ cup sunflower seed butter

¼ cup unsweetened rice, hemp, oat, or flax milk (check the ingredient list for any potential foods not allowed during the elimination phase)

1½ cups rolled oats (certified gluten-free)

½ teaspoon kosher salt

1. Line a rimmed baking sheet with parchment or wax paper.

2. In a large saucepan, bring the sugar, sunflower seed butter, and milk to a boil, stirring constantly; allow to boil for 1 minute. Remove from the heat and stir in the oats and salt.

3. Drop spoonfuls of the mixture onto the prepared baking sheet. Let cool and harden for about 30 minutes. Serve and enjoy.

STORAGE: Store in an airtight container in the refrigerator for up to 3 days or in the freezer for up to a month.

PER SERVING (1 MEDIUM COOKIE):
Calories: 199; Total fat: 9g; Total carbs: 27g; Fiber: 2g; Sugar: 18g; Protein: 5g; Sodium: 162mg

Banana-Apple Buckwheat Muffins

PREP TIME: 10 MINUTES | COOK TIME: 30 MINUTES | YIELD: 6 MUFFINS

Buckwheat is a naturally gluten-free flour that serves as the base for these muffins. I love making muffins, then storing them in the freezer for mornings when I'm in a hurry. These also make a delicious snack!

¼ cup buckwheat flour

½ teaspoon baking soda

⅛ teaspoon kosher salt

2 flax eggs (see page 85)

¼ cup cane sugar

½ banana, mashed

½ apple, cored and finely diced

1. Preheat the oven to 350°F. Line 6 cups of a standard muffin pan with paper liners.

2. In a small bowl, whisk together the flour, baking soda, and salt. In a medium bowl, combine the flax eggs, sugar, and banana. Add the dry ingredients to the wet and mix just until combined. Gently fold in the apple.

3. Pour the batter into the lined muffin cups. Bake for about 30 minutes, until a tester inserted in the center of a muffin comes out clean. Allow to cool on a rack.

STORAGE: Store in an airtight container at room temperature for up to 2 days, in the refrigerator for up to a week, or in the freezer for up to a month.

PER SERVING (1 MUFFIN): Calories: 74; Total fat: 1g; Total carbs: 16g; Fiber: 2g; Sugar: 11g; Protein: 1g; Sodium: 154mg

Blueberry Bread

PREP TIME: 10 MINUTES | COOK TIME: 1 HOUR 15 MINUTES | YIELD: 10 SLICES

This sweet bread resembles coffee cake, but using oat flour makes it naturally gluten-free and filled with fiber. I love eating this bread as part of a breakfast or even as a sweet treat at the end of a meal.

Canola oil cooking spray

2 cups rolled oats (certified gluten-free), ground in a food processor to a flour-like texture

1/2 cup cane sugar

1 teaspoon cream of tartar

1/2 teaspoon baking soda

1/2 teaspoon kosher salt

1 cup unsweetened rice, hemp, oat, or flax milk (check the ingredient list for any potential foods not allowed during the elimination phase)

3 tablespoons canola oil

1 1/2 cups fresh or frozen blueberries

1. Preheat the oven to 350°F. Spritz a 9-by-5-inch loaf pan with cooking spray.

2. In a large bowl, whisk together the oat flour, sugar, cream of tartar, baking soda, and salt.

3. In a small bowl, mix together the milk and oil. Add this to the dry ingredients and mix thoroughly. Gently fold in the blueberries.

4. Pour the batter into the prepared loaf pan and bake for 45 minutes. Turn off the oven and allow the bread to sit in the oven for 30 minutes before removing.

STORAGE: Store in an airtight container in the freezer for up to a month.

PER SERVING (1 SLICE): Calories: 151; Total fat: 6g; Total carbs: 25g; Fiber: 3g; Sugar: 12g; Protein: 2g; Sodium: 194mg

Creamy Mango Lassi

PREP TIME: 5 MINUTES | YIELD: 2 SERVINGS

A lassi is a traditional Indian beverage made with a yogurt base and sometimes fruit. This recipe puts a spin on a cold and creamy mango lassi I enjoyed years ago by swapping in nondairy milk for the yogurt and adding a touch of hemp seeds for extra healthy fat and plant protein. Cardamom is a spice that really makes this drink taste authentic.

1 frozen banana, cut into chunks

1½ cups frozen mango chunks

1½ cups unsweetened rice, hemp, oat, or flax milk (check the ingredient list for any potential foods not allowed during the elimination phase)

1 tablespoon hemp seeds

2 teaspoons maple or agave syrup

1 teaspoon minced or grated peeled fresh ginger

½ teaspoon ground cardamom

Combine all the ingredients in a heavy-duty blender and blend until smooth and creamy.

PER SERVING: Calories: 223; Total fat: 4g; Total carbs: 49g; Fiber: 9g; Sugar: 29g; Protein: 4g; Sodium: 106mg

Super-Seedy Crackers

PREP TIME: 5 MINUTES | COOK TIME: 1 HOUR | YIELD: ABOUT 24 LARGE CRACKERS

These crackers are made with chia, sunflower, and hemp seeds, giving them a nice crunch and texture. Chia is known for its healthy fat and fiber content, sunflower seeds are high in selenium and vitamin E, which act as antioxidants in the body, and hemp is a good source of healthy fats and protein. Enjoy these crackers all on their own or as a dipper for Garlic-Dill White Bean Dip (page 174).

1 cup chia seeds

1 cup shelled unsalted sunflower seeds (if you can find only salted, make sure there are no other ingredients that may cause a reaction, and adjust the salt as needed in the recipe)

1/2 cup hemp seeds

1 cup water

1 garlic clove, minced or grated

1/4 teaspoon plus a pinch kosher salt, divided

1. Preheat the oven to 300°F. Line a rimmed baking sheet with parchment paper or a silicone baking mat.

2. In a large bowl, combine all the seeds and stir until combined. Add the water, garlic, and 1/4 teaspoon of salt. Let this mixture sit for 2 minutes so the chia seeds can absorb the water.

3. Spread the mixture on the prepared baking sheet into two rectangles or ovals no more than 1/4 inch thick. Sprinkle a pinch of salt on top. Bake for 35 minutes.

4. Remove from the oven and carefully flip each cracker over. Bake for about 25 minutes more, until the edges begin to lightly brown.

5. Remove from the oven and let cool for 15 minutes on the pan. Break or cut into individual crackers and let cool the rest of the way on the pan.

STORAGE: Store in an airtight container at room temperature for up to 2 weeks or in the freezer for up to 1 month.

PER SERVING (1 CRACKER): Calories: 90; Total fat: 6g; Total carbs: 5g; Fiber: 4g; Sugar: 0g; Protein: 4g; Sodium: 25mg

Garlic-Dill White Bean Dip

This dip is similar to hummus and goes perfectly with some of your favorite chopped fresh vegetables or with Super-Seedy Crackers (page 173). Creamy, fresh, and flavorful—this will be a favorite snack in no time.

1 (15-ounce) can white beans, rinsed and drained

¼ cup unsweetened sunflower seed butter

3 garlic cloves, minced

1 teaspoon kosher salt

¼ cup canola oil

½ cup water

½ cup chopped fresh dill

1. Purée the beans, sunflower seed butter, garlic, and salt in a food processor until smooth. Scrape down the sides as necessary. With the machine running, pour the oil through the feed tube and process until thickened.

2. Add 1 tablespoon of water at a time until the consistency resembles that of hummus. Add the dill and pulse a few times to mix it in.

STORAGE: Store in an airtight container in the refrigerator for up to 5 days.

PER SERVING (2 TABLESPOONS):
Calories: 102; Total fat: 7g; Total carbs: 6g; Fiber: 2g; Sugar: 1g; Protein: 3g; Sodium: 214mg

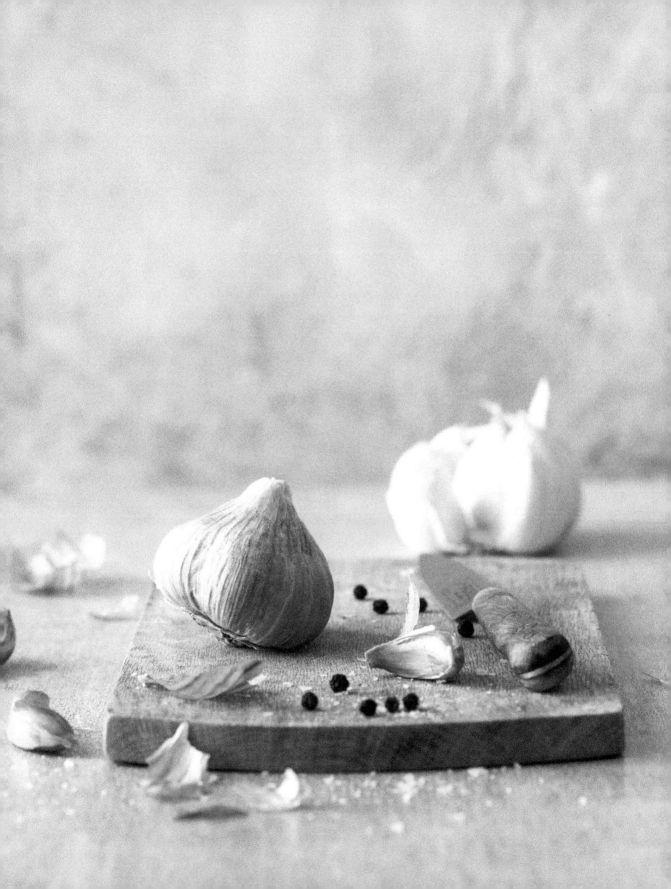

The Dirty Dozen™ and The Clean Fifteen™

A nonprofit environmental watchdog organization called the Environmental Working Group (EWG) looks at data supplied by the US Department of Agriculture (USDA) and the Food and Drug Administration (FDA) about pesticide residues. Each year, it compiles a list of the best and worst pesticide loads found in commercial crops. You can use these lists to decide which fruits and vegetables to buy organic to minimize your exposure to pesticides and which produce is considered safe enough to buy conventionally. This does not mean they are pesticide-free, though, so wash these fruits and vegetables thoroughly. The list is updated annually, and you can find it online at EWG.org/FoodNews.

Dirty Dozen™

1.	strawberries	5.	apples	9.	pears
2.	spinach	6.	grapes	10.	tomatoes
3.	kale	7.	peaches	11.	celery
4.	nectarines	8.	cherries	12.	potatoes

†Additionally, nearly three-quarters of hot pepper samples contained pesticide residues.

Clean Fifteen™

1.	avocados	6.	papayas	11.	cauliflower
2.	sweet corn	7.	eggplants	12.	cantaloupes
3.	pineapples	8.	asparagus	13.	broccoli
4.	sweet peas (frozen)	9.	kiwis	14.	mushrooms
5.	onions	10.	cabbages	15.	honeydew melons

Measurement Conversions

Volume Equivalents (Liquid)

US Standard	US Standard (ounces)	Metric (approximate)
2 tablespoons	1 fl. oz.	30 mL
¼ cup	2 fl. oz.	60 mL
½ cup	4 fl. oz.	120 mL
1 cup	8 fl. oz.	240 mL
1½ cups	12 fl. oz.	355 mL
2 cups or 1 pint	16 fl. oz.	475 mL
4 cups or 1 quart	32 fl. oz.	1 L
1 gallon	128 fl. oz.	4 L

Oven Temperatures

Fahrenheit	Celsius (approximate)
250°F	120°C
300°F	150°C
325°F	165°C
350°F	180°C
375°F	190°C
400°F	200°C
425°F	220°C
450°F	230°C

Volume Equivalents (Dry)

US Standard	Metric (approximate)
⅛ teaspoon	0.5 mL
¼ teaspoon	1 mL
½ teaspoon	2 mL
¾ teaspoon	4 mL
1 teaspoon	5 mL
1 tablespoon	15 mL
¼ cup	59 mL
⅓ cup	79 mL
½ cup	118 mL
⅔ cup	156 mL
¾ cup	177 mL
1 cup	235 mL
2 cups or 1 pint	475 mL
3 cups	700 mL
4 cups or 1 quart	1 L

Weight Equivalents

US Standard	Metric (approximate)
½ ounce	15 g
1 ounce	30 g
2 ounces	60 g
4 ounces	115 g
8 ounces	225 g
12 ounces	340 g
16 ounces or 1 pound	455 g

Resources

TaraRochfordNutrition.com

Food Allergy Research & Education: FoodAllergy.org

Food Allergies in Schools: CDC.gov/healthyschools/foodallergies/index.htm

Food Allergy vs. Food Intolerance: What's the Difference? MayoClinic.org /diseases-conditions/food-allergy/expert-answers/food-allergy/faq-20058538

Food Allergy: MayoClinic.org/diseases-conditions/food-allergy/symptoms -causes/syc-20355095

Food Allergies: Understanding Food Labels: MayoClinic.org/diseases-conditions /food-allergy/in-depth/food-allergies/art-20045949

Living with Food Allergies: KidsWithFoodAllergies.org/page/living-with-food -allergies.aspx

American College of Allergy, Asthma & Immunology: ACAAI.org

References

Introduction

Food Allergy Research & Education. "What Is a Food Allergy?" Accessed June 3, 2019. https://www.foodallergy.org/life-with-food-allergies/food-allergy-101/what-is-a-food-allergy.

World Allergy Organization. "World Allergy Week 2019 Will Focus on Food Allergy as a Global Problem." Last modified April 12, 2019. https://www.worldallergy.org/UserFiles/file/WorldAllergyWeek2019Announcementtopost.pdf.

Collins, Sherry Coleman. "Practice Paper of the Academy of Nutrition and Dietetics: Role of the Registered Dietitian Nutritionist in the Diagnosis and Management of Food Allergies." *Journal of the Academy of Nutrition and Dietetics* 116, no. 10 (October 2016): 1621–31. https://doi.org/10.1016/j.jand.2016.07.018.

Joneja, Janice. *The Health Professional's Guide to Food Allergies and Intolerances.* Academy of Nutrition and Dietetics, 2013.

Chapter 1: Food Allergies

Collins, Sherry Coleman. "Practice Paper of the Academy of Nutrition and Dietetics: Role of the Registered Dietitian Nutritionist in the Diagnosis and Management of Food Allergies." *Journal of the Academy of Nutrition and Dietetics* 116, no. 10 (October 2016): 1621–31. https://doi.org/10.1016/j.jand.2016.07.018.

Mayo Clinic. "Food Allergy." Last modified May 2, 2017. https://www.mayoclinic.org/diseases-conditions/food-allergy/symptoms-causes/syc-20355095.

Høst, Arne. "Frequency of Cow's Milk Allergy in Childhood." *Annals of Allergy, Asthma & Immunology* 89, no. 6 (December 2002): 33–7. https://doi.org/10.1016/S1081-1206(10)62120-5.

Mayo Clinic. "Milk Allergy." Last modified June 6, 2018. https://www.mayoclinic.org/diseases-conditions/milk-allergy/symptoms-causes/syc-20375101.

Mayo Clinic. "Wheat Allergy." Last modified May 5, 2018. https://www.mayoclinic.org/diseases-conditions/wheat-allergy/symptoms-causes/syc-20378897.

Pastorello, Elide A. et al. "Wheat IgE-Mediated Food Allergy in European Patients: α-Amylase Inhibitors, Lipid Transfer Proteins and Low-Molecular-Weight Glutenins." *International Archives of Allergy and Immunology* 144, no. 1 (August 2007): 10–22. https://doi.org/10.1159/000102609.

Joneja, Janice. *The Health Professional's Guide to Food Allergies and Intolerances*. Academy of Nutrition and Dietetics, 2013.

Sicherer, S., and H. Sampson. "Food Allergy." *Journal of Allergy and Clinical Immunology* 117, no. 2 (February 2006): S470–5. https://doi.org/10.1016/j.jaci.2005.05.048.

Mayo Clinic. "Egg Allergy." Last modified May 7, 2019. https://www.mayoclinic.org/diseases-conditions/egg-allergy/symptoms-causes/syc-20372115.

Sicherer, Scott H. et al. "Prevalence of Seafood Allergy in the United States Determined by a Random Telephone Survey." *Journal of Allergy and Clinical Immunology* 114, no. 1 (July 2004): 159–65. https://doi.org/10.1016/j.jaci.2004.04.018.

Hamada, Yuki et al. "Identification of Collagen as a New Fish Allergen." *Bioscience, Biotechnology, and Biochemistry* 65, no. 2 (2001): 285–91. https://doi.org/10.1271/bbb.65.285.

American College of Allergy, Asthma & Immunology. "Fish Allergy." Last modified March 21, 2019. https://acaai.org/allergies/types/food-allergies/types-food-allergy/fish-allergy.

Mayo Clinic. "Shellfish Allergy." Last modified April 13, 2019. https://www.mayoclinic.org/diseases-conditions/shellfish-allergy/symptoms-causes/syc-20377503.

Mayo Clinic. "Soy Allergy." Last modified April 11, 2018. https://www.mayoclinic.org /diseases-conditions/soy-allergy/symptoms-causes/syc-20377802.

Al-Muhsen, Saleh et al. "Peanut Allergy: An Overview." *Canadian Medical Association Journal* 168, no. 10 (May 2003): 1279–85. http://www.cmaj.ca/content/cmaj/168/10 /1279.full.pdf.

Mayo Clinic. "Peanut Allergy." Last modified November 13, 2018. https://www .mayoclinic.org/diseases-conditions/peanut-allergy/symptoms-causes/syc-20376175.

American College of Allergy, Asthma & Immunology. "Tree Nut Allergy." Accessed November 2, 2018. https://acaai.org/allergies/types/food-allergies/types-food-allergy /tree-nut-allergy.

Sicherer, Scott H. et al. "US Prevalence of Self-Reported Peanut, Tree Nut, and Sesame Allergy: 11-Year Follow-Up." *Journal of Allergy and Clinical Immunology* 125, no. 6 (June 2010): 1322–6. https://doi.org/10.1016/j.jaci.2010.03.029.

Government of Canada. "Sesame: A Priority Food Allergen." Last modified August 31, 2016. https://www.canada.ca/en/health-canada/services/food-nutrition/reports -publications/food-safety/sesame-priority-food-allergen.html.

Food Allergy Research & Education. "Sesame Allergy." Accessed May 2, 2019. https://www.foodallergy.org/common-allergens/sesame-allergy.

American College of Allergy, Asthma & Immunology. "Corn Allergy." Last modified March 8, 2019. https://acaai.org/allergies/types/food-allergies/types-food-allergy /corn-allergy.

American College of Allergy, Asthma & Immunology. "Oral Allergy Syndrome." Last modified March 21, 2019. https://acaai.org/allergies/types/food-allergies/types-food -allergy/oral-allergy-syndrome.

Ebner, C. et al. "Identification of Allergens in Fruits and Vegetables: IgE Cross-Reactivities with the Important Birch Pollen Allergens Bet v 1 and Bet v 2 (Birch Profilin)." *Journal of Allergy and Clinical Immunology* 95, no. 5 (1995): 962–9. https://doi.org/10.1016/s0091-6749(95)70096-x.

Kim, Jung-Hyun et al. "Oral Allergy Syndrome in Birch Pollen-Sensitized Patients from a Korean University Hospital." *Journal of Korean Medical Science* 33, no. 33 (2018). https://doi.org/10.3346/jkms.2018.33.e218.

Kondo, Yasuto, and Atsuo Urisu. "Oral Allergy Syndrome." *Allergology International* 58, no. 4 (2009): 485–91. https://doi.org/10.2332/allergolint.09-RAI-0136.

Wagner, S., and H. Breiteneder. "The Latex-Fruit Syndrome." *Biochemical Society Transactions* 30, no. 6 (2002): 935–40. https://doi.org/10.1042/bst0300935.

Blanco, Carlos. "Latex-Fruit Syndrome." *Current Allergy and Asthma Reports* 3, no. 1 (2003): 47–53. https://doi.org/10.1007/s11882-003-0012-y.

Hosey, Robert G., Peter J. Carek, and Alvin Goo. "Exercise-Induced Anaphylaxis and Urticaria." *American Family Physician* 64, no. 8 (October 15, 2001): 1367–73.

Chapter 2: Food Intolerances and Sensitivities

Joneja, Janice. *The Health Professional's Guide to Food Allergies and Intolerances.* Academy of Nutrition and Dietetics, 2013.

Mahan, L. Kathleen, and Janice L. Raymond. *Krause's Food & the Nutrition Care Process.* Saunders, 2017.

Mayo Clinic. "Gluten-Free Diet." Last modified November 23, 2017. https://www.mayoclinic.org/healthy-lifestyle/nutrition-and-healthy-eating/in-depth/gluten-free-diet/art-20048530.

Celiac Disease Foundation. "What Is Gluten?" Accessed May 8, 2019. https://celiac.org/gluten-free-living/what-is-gluten/.

Celiac Disease Foundation. "What Is Celiac Disease?" Accessed May 8, 2019. https://celiac.org/about-celiac-disease/what-is-celiac-disease/.

Uhde, Melanie et al. "Intestinal Cell Damage and Systemic Immune Activation in Individuals Reporting Sensitivity to Wheat in the Absence of Coeliac Disease." *Gut* 65, no. 12 (2016): 1930–7. https://doi.org/10.1136/gutjnl-2016-311964.

Bosnir, Danijel Brkic Jasna et al. "Nitrate in Leafy Green Vegetables and Estimated Intake." *African Journal of Traditional, Complementary and Alternative Medicines* 14, no. 3 (2017): 31–41. https://doi.org/10.21010/ajtcam.v14i3.4.

Hord, Norman G. et al. "Food Sources of Nitrates and Nitrites: The Physiologic Context for Potential Health Benefits." *American Journal of Clinical Nutrition* 90, no. 1 (2009): 1–10. https://doi.org/10.3945/ajcn.2008.27131.

Maintz, Laura, and Natalija Novak. "Histamine and Histamine Intolerance." *American Journal of Clinical Nutrition* 85, no. 5 (2007): 1185–96. https://doi.org/10.1093/ajcn/85.5.1185.

Joneja, Janice. *The Beginner's Guide to Histamine Intolerance.* Berrydales Books, 2017.

Tarasoff, L., and M. F. Kelly. "Monosodium L-Glutamate: A Double-Blind Study and Review." *Food and Chemical Toxicology* 31, no. 12 (1993): 1019–35. https://doi.org/10.1016/0278-6915(93)90012-n.

Chapman, Jean et al. "Food Allergy: A Practice Parameter." *Pediatric Allergy: Principles and Practice* 96 (March 2006): S1–68.

Lester, M R. "Sulfite Sensitivity: Significance in Human Health." *Journal of the American College of Nutrition* 14, no. 3 (1995): 229–32. https://doi.org/10.1080/07315724.1995.10718500.

Vally, Hassan, and Niel LA Masso. "Adverse Reactions to the Sulphite Additives." *Gastroenterology and Hepatology from Bed to Bench* 5, no. 1 (2012): 16–23.

Kajiyama, Hiroshi et al. "Elevated Levels of Serum Sulfite in Patients with Chronic Renal Failure." *Journal of the American Society of Nephrology* 11, no. 5 (May 1, 2000): 923–7.

"Final Report on the Safety Assessment of Benzyl Alcohol, Benzoic Acid, and Sodium Benzoate." *International Journal of Toxicology* 20, no. 3 (2001): 23–50. https://doi.org/10.1080/10915810152630729.

Pacor, M. L. et al. "Monosodium Benzoate Hypersensitivity in Subjects with Persistent Rhinitis." *Allergy* 59, no. 2 (2004): 192–7. https://doi.org/10.1046/j.1398-9995.2003.00380.x.

Arnold, L. Eugene et al. "Artificial Food Colors and Attention-Deficit/Hyperactivity Symptoms: Conclusions to Dye For." *Neurotherapeutics* 9, no. 3 (2012): 599–609. https://doi.org/10.1007/s13311-012-0133-x.

Dipalma, JR. "Tartrazine Sensitivity." *American Family Physician* 42, no. 5 (November 1990): 1347–50.

Ros, Ann-Mari et al. "A Follow-up Study of Patients with Recurrent Urticaria and Hypersensitivity to Aspirin, Benzoates and Azo Dyes." *British Journal of Dermatology* 95, no. 1 (1976): 19–24. https://doi.org/10.1111/j.1365-2133.1976.tb15532.x.

Bateman, B. "The Effects of a Double Blind, Placebo Controlled, Artificial Food Colourings and Benzoate Preservative Challenge on Hyperactivity in a General Population Sample of Preschool Children." *Archives of Disease in Childhood* 89, no. 6 (2004): 506–11. https://doi.org/10.1136/adc.2003.031435.

Yang, Amy et al. "Genetics of Caffeine Consumption and Responses to Caffeine." *Psychopharmacology* 211, no. 3 (2010): 245–57. https://doi.org/10.1007/s00213-010-1900-1.

Sugiyama, Kumiya et al. "Anaphylaxis Due to Caffeine." *Asia Pacific Allergy* 5, no. 1 (2015): 55. https://doi.org/10.5415/apallergy.2015.5.1.55.

Chapter 3: Diagnosing Food Allergies and Sensitivities

Collins, Sherry Coleman. "Practice Paper of the Academy of Nutrition and Dietetics: Role of the Registered Dietitian Nutritionist in the Diagnosis and Management of Food Allergies." *Journal of the Academy of Nutrition and Dietetics* 116, no. 10 (October 2016): 1621–31. https://doi.org/10.1016/j.jand.2016.07.018.

"Guidelines for the Diagnosis and Management of Food Allergy in the United States: Report of the NIAID-Sponsored Expert Panel." *Journal of Allergy and Clinical Immunology* 126, no. 6 (2010). https://doi.org/10.1016/j.jaci.2010.10.007.

Fleischer, David M., and A. Wesley Burks. "Pitfalls in Food Allergy Diagnosis: Serum IgE Testing." *Journal of Pediatrics* 166, no. 1 (2015): 8–10. https://doi.org/10.1016/j.jpeds.2014.09.057.

Food Allergy Research & Education. "Skin Prick Tests." Accessed May 8, 2019. https://www.foodallergy.org/life-with-food-allergies/food-allergy-101/diagnosis-testing/skin-prick-tests.

Chapter 4: The Elimination Phase

Sampson, Hugh A. "Food Allergy. Part 2: Diagnosis and Management." *Journal of Allergy and Clinical Immunology* 103, no. 6 (1999): 981–9. https://doi.org/10.1016/S0091-6749(99)70167-3.

Joneja, Janice. *The Beginner's Guide to Histamine Intolerance.* Berrydale's Books, 2017.

Joneja, Janice. *The Health Professional's Guide to Food Allergies and Intolerances.* Academy of Nutrition and Dietetics, 2013.

Hord, Norman G. et al. "Food Sources of Nitrates and Nitrites: The Physiologic Context for Potential Health Benefits." *American Journal of Clinical Nutrition* 90, no. 1 (2009): 1–10. https://doi.org/10.3945/ajcn.2008.27131.

"Electronic Code of Federal Regulations." Accessed May 2, 2019. https://www.ecfr.gov/cgi-bin/text-idx?c=ecfr&SID=0f29870bbafc6ae3d1efc78d9927d918&tpl=%2Fecfrbrowse%2FTitle21%2F21cfr73_main_02.tpl.

U.S. Food & Drug Administration. "Food Allergen Labeling and Consumer Protection Act of 2004 (FALCPA)." Accessed April 20, 2019. https://www.fda.gov/food/food-allergens-and-gluten-free-guidance-documents-and-regulatory-information/food-allergen-labeling-and-consumer-protection-act-2004-falcpa.

"Guidelines for the Diagnosis and Management of Food Allergy in the United States: Report of the NIAID-Sponsored Expert Panel." *Journal of Allergy and Clinical Immunology* 126, no. 6 (2010). https://doi.org/10.1016/j.jaci.2010.10.007.

Food Allergy Research & Education. "Milk Allergy." Accessed May 2, 2019. https://www.foodallergy.org/common-allergens/milk-allergy.

Food Allergy Research & Education. "Egg Allergy." Accessed May 2, 2019. https://www.foodallergy.org/common-allergens/egg-allergy.

Food Allergy Research & Education. "Soy Allergy." Accessed May 2, 2019. https://www.foodallergy.org/common-allergens/soy-allergy.

Food Allergy Research & Education. "Sesame Allergy." Accessed May 2, 2019. https://www.foodallergy.org/common-allergens/sesame-allergy.

Patriarca, G. et al. "Food Allergy and Food Intolerance: Diagnosis and Treatment." *Internal and Emergency Medicine* 4, no. 1 (February 2009): 11–24. https://doi.org/10.1007/s11739-008-0183-6.

Joneja, Janice. *The Health Professional's Guide to Food Allergies and Intolerances.* Academy of Nutrition and Dietetics, 2013.

Sicherer, S. H. "Food Allergy: When and How to Perform Oral Food Challenges." *Pediatric Allergy and Immunology* 10, no. 4 (January 2002): 226–34. https://doi.org/10.1034/j.1399-3038.1999.00040.x.

Index

reintroduction phase, 23, 47–55

Enzyme-linked immunosorbent assay (ELISA), 22

F

Fats, 30

Fish, 33, 52

Fish allergies, 6

Flax eggs, 85

Fluorescent allergosorbent test (FAST), 22

Food Allergen Labeling and Consumer Protection Act (FALCPA), 40

Food allergies. *See also specific allergies*

defined, 3

diagnosing, 21–23

symptoms, 3–4, 51

Food-dependent exercise-induced anaphylaxis (FDEIA), 5, 10

Food journal, 49–50

Food sensitivities/intolerances, 14

Freezer Chicken Meatballs, 126

Fresh Greens and Blueberry Salad with Easy Dill Dressing, 76

Fruits, 28. *See also specific*

G

Garlic-Dill White Bean Dip, 174

Garlic-Ginger Bok Choy, 159

Garlic-Roasted Broccoli, 154

Garlic Skillet Chicken, 119

Ginger

Back Pocket Stir-Fry with Rice Noodles, 123–124

Beef and Broccoli Bowl, 132–133

Creamy Mango Lassi, 172

Egg Roll Bowls, 142

Garlic-Ginger Bok Choy, 159

Mango Oat Crumble Bars, 168

Slow Cooker Maple-Garlic Chicken, 109

Slow Cooker Pork Stir-Fry, 146–147

Superfood Salad, 73–74

Sweet Potato Buddha Bowl, 82–83

Sweet Potato Zoodle Soup with Creamy Turmeric Sauce, 102

Gluten, 14, 36, 52

Gluten intolerance, 15

Golden Roasted Cauliflower and Brown Rice Salad, 68–69

Grains/starches, 29

Greek Meatball Salad, 148–149

H

Hemp seeds

Banana Oatmeal with Hemp and Chia Seeds, 61

Blueberry Breakfast Smoothie, 64

Chicken Skewers with Basil Pesto, 121–122

Creamy Mango Lassi, 172

Greek Meatball Salad, 148–149

Mediterranean Mason Jar Pesto Salad, 78–79

Roasted Vegetable and Brown Rice Bowl with Green Sauce, 80–81

Spaghetti Squash and Meatballs, 136–137

Spring Roll Bowl, 90–91

Super-Seedy Crackers, 173

Sweet Potato Falafel Bowl, 84–85

Tropical Green Smoothie, 65

Herbal teas, 31

Herbs, 30. *See also specific*

Herby Cauliflower Salad, 75

Herby Pork Meatballs with Roasted Apples, 143

Histamines, 16, 36–37, 42, 54

I

Immunoglobulin A (IgA), 14

Immunoglobulin E (IgE), 4, 14

Ingredient labels, 40–43

Italian Chicken Burgers with Roasted Vegetables, 127–128

K

Kale

Bell Pepper and Basil Wild Rice Bowl, 86

Blueberry-Basil Mason Jar Salad, 77

Chicken Soup with Quinoa and Greens, 97–98

About the Author

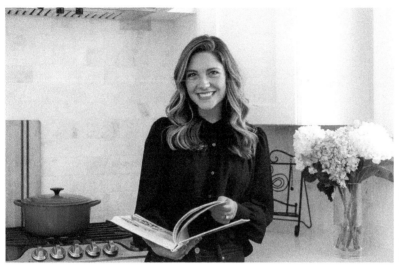

© Kelley Jordan Schuyler

Tara Rochford, RDN, is a registered dietitian, recipe developer, healthy living blogger, and dog mom. She writes at TaraRochfordNutrition.com, a website where she shares simple and delicious recipes, science-backed nutrition information, and tips for helping individuals find their version of healthy. It is her mission to share with the world that nourishing foods are delicious and comforting for the soul and should never be tasteless or bland.

Tara has worked as the registered dietitian for Butler University, currently teaches nutritious cooking classes in the Indianapolis community, and has a monthly cooking segment on the local lifestyle show *Indy Style*.

Tara lives in Indianapolis with her husband and two vizslas, Bernie and Rooney. In her spare time, she enjoys exploring the world through food, training for half marathons, and cuddling with her Velcro vizslas.